About the author......

Late Dr. Ramesh Mathur, former Professor of Zoology, Director-College of Pharmacy and Director-Department of Neuroscience Jiwaji University, Gwalior, was credited to have 40 years' experience in teaching and research. He published 220 research papers in national and international research journals and 15 books including three reference books. 64 students obtained Ph.D. degree under his guidance. He conduced 12 research projects sanctioned by various agencies like U.G.C., I.C.M.R., D.R.D.O., Ministry of Environment and Forests and M.P.C.S.T. He was well known in the field of Reproductive Biology and Toxicology. Having administrative experience of about fifteen years, Dr. Mathur had contributed immensely in starting new courses and organizing various conferences and edited Asian Journal of Experimental Sciences.

ABOUT THE BOOK....

While heart disease declined 60 percent in the last 30 years in the United States, it has escalated by 300 percent in India. Indian men, no matter where they live, have one of the highest rates of heart disease in the world, even if they have low levels of traditional risk factors such as cholesterol. Each year about 15 Lac Indians die due to coronary heart disease. In fact, even non-smoking vegetarians under 40 who exercise regularly may be at high risk. While 60 percent of heart attacks amongst Americans occur after the age 55, nearly half of all heart attacks among Indian men strike under the age of 55 and 25 percent under the age of 40. Indian women also share these high rates of heart disease. A growing number of young urban Indians are now being afflicted. Children as young as 10 have fatty deposits and people as young as 20 have plaque formation in the arteries.

Fatty diet is one of the major causes of heart disease. People need to be made aware and motivated to adopt diet suitable for keeping the heart fit. There is confusion about the quality of different cooking oils. It is attempted to outline the properties of common cooking oils to make it convenient to select the one suitable to the heart and the individual pocket. Beneficial effects of some food items have also been highlighted.

An inactive life enhances the risk of heart problem, therefore proper exercises and how much one should exercise has been described.

Sleep has a direct relationship with the occurrence of heart and other health problems. Repercussions and the ways to have sound sleep have been dealt with.

Hospitalization is a major demoralizing event for the patient and his care takers, who need to be educated to be ready about the program in the hospital and the time there after.

There exist malpractices in medical profession, as is evident by the cases exposed time to time. The patients are misguided and made to incur unnecessary expenditure. They should be aware of the various diseases of the heart and the techniques involved in their treatment.

The book also deals with some other aspects, which are important for prevention and cure of heart problems.

CONTENT

PREFACE

While heart disease declined 60 percent in the last 30 years in the United States, it has escalated by 300 percent in India. U.S. studies have found that Indians in the United States have three to four times the heart disease rate of the mainstream U.S. population. Another study by the HMO Kaiser Permanente in California found that hospitalization rates for heart surgery among Indian Americans are four times that of the Americans. Indian men, no matter where they live, have one of the highest rates of heart disease in the world, even if they have low levels of traditional risk factors such as cholesterol. In fact, even non-smoking vegetarians under 40 who exercise regularly may be at high risk. While 60 percent of heart attacks amongst Americans occur after age 55, nearly half of all heart attacks among Indian men strike under the age of 55 and 25 percent under the age of 40. Indian women also share these high rates of heart disease. Thousands of Indian American men in their 40s and 50s succumb to a first, fatal heart attack every year. "Every population gets heart disease and diabetes, but Indians get more of it and gets it at least ten years earlier," says Dr.Enas A. Enas, Director of the Coronary Artery Disease among Asian Indians Research Foundation at the University of Illinois at Chicago.

In late eighties of the last century, it was prophesied by the world cardiologists that in future the cardiac surgery will be almost bloodless. Heart disease being number one killer, this was taken as a big news. Till date heart patients are waiting and asking worrisome questions. The assurance given is yet to be fulfilled. The cardiac surgery is not yet bloodless; however, there are some options before going for operation. In past the person did not know about the disease until he suffered. Today improved screening techniques like CAT scanning, MRI PET scan, Stress cardiography and other tests educate us abut the problem and the treatment before having a heart attack. Even if there is a problem in coronary artery one need not to go for open heart surgery. Angioplasty, a less invasive surgery can compress the plaque and open the artery. In initial stages angioplasty seemed to be fifty percent failure as patients had their vessels reclogged after six months or one year. Use of stent- a wire -mesh tube inserted into the problematic artery has made angioplasty the top treatment against blocking arteries as it supports it against collapsing. "I did around 200 bypass surgeries a year when I started operating in Mumbai in 1992," says Dr Ramakanta Panda, AHI's Chief Executive Officer and consultant cardio-thoracic surgeon." This increased to 500 in a few years, and now I do a thousand." Last year in India, surgeons performed some 55,000 coronary bypass operations.

A few decades ago, Indians had plenty of physical activity and ate lots of grains and vegetables and very little saturated fats, so they were considered immune to coronary heart disease. Now it is not like that. Coronary heart disease is one of the leading causes of death in India. 16.5 percent of all male deaths and 17.1 of all female deaths are due to CHD. Many of the factors for growth of this killer disease include unhealthy diet, low physical activity and stressful life. Moreover, a high fat diet and obesity contribute in rise of cholesterol and blood fats which obstruct free flow of blood in the coronary arteries. WHO estimates that in coming years India will have 100 million people suffering from heart disease. Unlike in the West where most of the patients suffer with one artery blockage, Indians have two or three artery blockages. It is not clear if it is a genetic disorder or a metabolic syndrome, but Indians are blamed to have unhealthy lifestyle causing high cholesterol and triglycerides levels. There is significant decrease in cardiovascular diseases in America, Canada and Australia, perhaps because of public education, treatment and screening programs and having a heart healthy life style.

In today's busy life people do not have time to think about their health problems and their causes. Whenever somebody feels discomfort, he takes home medicines without understanding what the symptoms suggest. If at all he goes to a doctor, just starts taking medicines. Patient should go to the doctor prepared with some questions regarding the problem. In India doctors have to examine many patients, so not always they find time to tell the details of the ailment. They just write the prescription and let the patient go. If the patient insists, the doctor discusses. It is necessary to know the cause so that suitable measures may be taken.

The problem is that most people decide to see a doctor when they experience a heart attack. They are rushed to a specialist hospital and saved. They are advised to control weight, take balanced diet and do regular exercise but why they undergo trauma is not understood and what type of life style they have and what may be the consequences. Better it is to learn and practice simpler methods for preventing cardiovascular problems. If one does not understand angina or angiography, he may be led to go for open heart surgery or the like. Experts say that most of the ailments give indications to the body. If we take them seriously, timely action may be taken.

No two people are exactly alike and they not necessarily respond to the treatment in the same way. People under treatment if understand their ailment they may help the doctor a lot. They get a positive mind set which is a powerful motivating force for better recovery

The present guide attempts to cover concisely a lot

of ground by linking the bits of information collected from internet, medical books and journals and popular magazines, as well as from the writer's personal experience as a heart patient.

FUNCTIONING OF THE HEART

The heart consists of two atria and two ventricles. Atria are separated by an interatrial septum and the ventricles by the interventricular septum. The right atrium receives deoxygenated blood from the body tissues and pours it into the right ventricle. The left atrium receives oxygenated blood from the lungs and pours it into the left ventricle. The left ventricle is larger than the right ventricle and has thick wall. The heart works day and night by alternate contraction (systole) and relaxation (diastole). The two atria begin their contraction at the same time and the blood from both the atria is poured into the respective ventricles. The back flow of the blood is prevented by the atrio-ventricular valves. Ventricles also contract simultaneously. The right ventricle forces the blood into the pulmonary aorta which takes it to the lungs for oxygenation, while the left ventricle forces blood into the systemic aorta which distributes it to all parts of the body.

SPECIALIZED CONDUCTING SYSTEM OF THE HEART

During embryonic development about one percent of the heart muscle fibers become auto rhythmic fibers. These relatively rare fibers have two important functions:

1.   They act as pace maker, setting rhythm of electric excitation that causes contraction of the heart muscle.

2.   They form the conduction system, a network of specialized cardiac muscle fibers that provide a path for each impulse of contraction to pass through the heart. The conduction system ensures that the cardiac chambers are stimulated to contract in a coordinated manner, which makes the heart to work like a pump. The cardiac stimulation propagates through the conduction system in the following sequence.

3.   The Sinoatrial node (S-A node) is a specialized portion of the heart which is capable of generating electrical impulse responsible for the propagation of the wave of contraction. It is present in the dorsal wall of the right atrium, near the entrance of the right superior vena cava in the right atrium. Cells of the S-A node do not have a stable resting potential, when the potential reaches a particular height, it is known as pace maker potential. It triggers an action potential throughout both the atria and the atria undergo contraction. The S-A node spontaneously produces

contractions at the rate of 60-100 beats per minute. This rate is constantly modified by the activity of sympathetic and parasympathetic nerves so that the resting cardiac rate in adult human is about 70 beats per minute. The sympathetic nerves increase the heart beat while parasympathetic nerves decrease the beat. Because the Sinoatrial node is responsible for the contraction of the rest of the heart, it is known as the Primary Pacemaker.

A-V junction Node and Bundle of His (Secondary Pace maker)

A-V node is located in the posterior part of the interatrial septum, just anterior to the opening of the coronary sinus. Its main function is to retain the impulse of contraction for a while till all the blood from atria is transferred to the ventricles. When S-A node is unable to transmit the impulse of contraction, the A-V node functions as the Secondary Pace maker. The cells of the A-V node discharge impulse of contraction at the rate of 40 to 60 beats per minute.

The A-V node continues into the Bundle of His. This bundle is the only place through which the stimulus of contraction can conduct from atria to the ventricles. Other places are insulated by the fibrous skeleton of the heart. After propagation through the bundle of His (A-V bundle) the wave of contraction enters the right and left branches of this bundle and the Purkinje fibers, which carries the wave to their respective areas. Purkinje fibers which have large diameter rapidly conduct the stimulus beginning at the apex of the heart upwards towards entire ventricular muscle. This results in contraction of the ventricle pushing blood towards the systemic aorta and the pulmonary aorta. These fibers can produce 30 to 40 beats per minute when S-A node and A-V node fail to function.

Normally the S-A node is the main structure producing impulse of contraction. The action potential generated by the S-A node passes down the cardiac conduction system and arrives before the other cells produce their spontaneous action potential.

CHEMICAL REGULATION OF THE HEART

Besides, the S-A node maintains the heart beat at normal rate, the sympathetic and parasympathetic nervous systems also regulate the heart rate. Epinephrine and nor epinephrine are the hormones released from the sympathetic nerves and adrenal medulla which increase the heart rate as well as contractility. Exercise, stress and excitement induce increased release of these hormones. Thyroid hormone also increases heart rate. Patients suffering from hyperthyroidism may have increased heart rate (tachycardia). Acetylcholine secreted by the parasympathetic nerves slows down the heart rate. Our body always remains under tone of either sympathetic or parasympathetic nervous system. When we are standing or sitting, the body is under sympathetic control while when we lie down parallel to the ground, the body comes under parasympathetic tone. It is because of this reason that when we sleep the heart rate and force of contraction is decreased. Most of the heart attacks occur in early morning hours when heart beat is slow and contractility is weak as a result of which blood does not pass through already obstructed coronary arteries.

OTHER FACTORS REGULATING THE HEART RATE

Age, gender, physical fitness and body temperature also influence resting heart rate. A new born baby has a resting heart rate over 120 beats per minute. The rate then gradually declines throughout the life span. Adult females have resting heart rate slightly slower than the males. A slowly beating heart is more energy efficient than that which beats rapidly. During fever or strenuous exercise, the body temperature rises and the heart beat increases. Decreased temperature decreases heart rate as well as force of contraction. During surgical repair the patient's heart is slowed down by cooling the patient's body too low so that the metabolism of the body is lowered which reduces the oxygen demand of the tissues and the heart and the brain have to work less and blood flow is reduced, thus facilitating the surgical procedure.

COMMON DISEASES OF THE HEART

The term heart disease includes the problems related to the heart and the blood vessels. There are many different types of heart diseases and each has its specific symptoms. Diseases of blood vessels are more common now a days and majority of deaths occur due to vascular problems like hypertension or coronary artery blockage. The following account gives information about some of the common diseases. One should be alert enough about any symptoms if they appear. This will give a healthy body and good quality of life.

The most common diseases of the heart include:

(1)   **Congenital malformations**

These are developmental defects of the heart from birth, a condition in which there may be some defect in the structure of the heart of the newborn. As a result of it there is variety of problems like blood not getting to the heart and blood vessels in normal giving rise to irregular pulse. The baby may have a hole in the partition of the heart. This causes wrong flow of blood and causes mixing of oxygenated and deoxygenated blood as a result of which the pure blood is not supplied to important body organs like brain which may lead to complications. The oxygenated blood is bright red in color while deoxygenated blood is bluish. This gives a bluish tinge to the baby and such a baby is known as blue baby. There may be other congenital defects also.

(2)   **Long   Q-T syndrome**

In this disorder the congenital heart defect remains dormant for years and sometime later in life it springs from nowhere and causes sudden fainting, ventricular fibrillation and even sudden death. Long Q-T syndrome may also be triggered by some type of excitement, exercise or sex.

(3) **Heart valve disease**

When heart valves do not open and close in the normal way, as a result of which the blood may accumulate at wrong places in the heart and the body organs do not get proper blood supply. This condition may be due to many factors including some types of cancers and chromosomal defects

There may be various causes of infection but more common are rheumatic fever, syphilis, and bacterial endocarditis. In rheumatic fever, the heart valves, the inner wall of the heart (endocardium) and muscle of the heart (myocardium) are affected. Most commonly it causes hardening of one of the valves- condition known as mitral stenosis. In endocarditis bacteria attach to the heart valve. Enough number of white blood cells does not reach them as these valves have poor blood supply. Due to availability of a number of antibiotics this can be controlled.

A large number of studies have associated heart disease with chronic bacterial and viral infections. In 1980 patients suffering from atherosclerosis were found to be infected with a number of bacteria like *Helicobactor pyroli, and Chlamydia pneumonie* and certain viruses particularly *cytomegalovirus.* In one study Petra Saikki and colleagues at the University of Helsinki, Finland found that 27 out of 40 patients who suffered heart attack and 15 out of 30 men with heart disease carried antibodies related to *Chlamydia,* which is more commonly known as gum disease. Compared to subjects who were free of heart disease, only 7 out of 41 had such antibodies. Researchers have found fragments of bacteria in arterial plaques. In developed countries many adult people suffer from the infection of above bacteria and virus. Presence of antibodies against these organisms does not necessarily mean that they are infected but it indicates that they were infected once upon a time. Mostly infection from these organisms persists indefinitely. Once infected with herpes, the virus remains for life. When the immune system weakens, the infection appears. When these microorganisms enter an artery, they can attack its wall with low grade infection without any noticeable symptoms. When they colonize the artery, they damage cells of the wall causing inflammation. To heal the injured blood platelets, cholesterol and protein set in at the site of damage and thus initiate the formation of the plaque. Besides microorganisms, factors like free radicals, high blood pressure and diabetes may also damage the arterial wall and cause plaque formation.

(4) Atrial Myxoma

In this condition the atrial septum which divides the two atria develops a noncancerous tumor.

Mostly it occurs on the right side and therefore, the right atrioventricular valve or the tricuspid valve is affected. The right atrioventricular opening is narrowed at its opening. As a result of this the filling of the right ventricle may remain incomplete and the lungs receive lesser blood for purification. It may also cause irregular heart beat (atrial fibrillation).

(5) Hypertrophic-Cardiomyopathy

In this disease muscles of the heart (myocardium) becomes thick for some unknown cause. This condition may cause sudden heart attack in people of any age group. This can be seen in athletes who are in good activity but may have surprise heart attack.

Excessive workload on the heart---This type of condition is caused when the heart has been put to stress for a long time as (1) in high blood pressure where left ventricle is subjected to considerable strain, (2) bronchial asthma or chronic bronchitis when right ventricle is put to stress and (3) valvular deformities, where both the ventricles are put to stress.

(6) Angina

When heart muscle does not get sufficient oxygen supply (ischemia), it gives chest pain. This is commonly called as angina. This is due to obstruction of the coronary arteries or their spasm. More common cause of angina is atherosclerosis*, a condition when plaque formation takes place inside the artery wall. There is a weak relationship between severity of pain in the chest and decrease in oxygen supply to the heart muscle. There can be severe pain with no risk of heart attack or there may be a heart attack without pain. Along with the chest pain the patient may experience pain in the inner left arm, shoulders and the jaws.

* Hardening & narrowing of the arteries caused by plaque build-up.
Pain may be associated with breathlessness, sweating and nausea in some cases.
It generally occurs by exertion or emotional stress. It is exacerbated by having a full stomach and extreme cold condition. Pulse rate and blood pressure may increase.
Angina may be:

(1)   **Stable angina**: It occurs with chest pain and associated symptoms after physical activity like walking or running. On rest the symptoms minimize or completely subside. It may again occur after activity.
(2)   **Unstable angina**: This is a form of acute coronary syndrome and is known as angina pectoris.

It may show one of the following features:
(i)   It occurs at rest or with little exertion.

(ii)   It is severe and occurs within 4 to 6 weeks of the onset of problem (ischemia).

(iii)   It is prolonged and more frequent.

Unstable angina is unpredictable as it may occur at rest; therefore, it is an indicator of an impending heart attack. It is caused due to reduced blood supply to the heart muscle as a result of platelet aggregation on the inner wall of the artery, coronary artery spasm or coronary thrombosis. 64% of unstable angina occurs between 10PM and 8AM. (Rest period) Instable angina the developing atheroma is protected by a cap. In unstable angina this cap is ruptured which allows blood clots to accumulate, reducing the lumen of the vessel. This explains why unstable angina may occur at rest.

(7) Increase in heart size

Sometime in cardiac patients the size of the heart increases which can be diagnosed by X-RAY. Despite enlargement in size the heart may supply sufficient blood to the body organs for a number of years. However, complications like pneumonia, loss of blood, over exertion or pregnancy may lead to heart failure. In case of athletes the heart is usually enlarged which may cause problems in nonactive post- retirement period?

Diseases of the heart are not found only in the aged individuals. The highest incidences are found between the ages of 40 to 60 years in western countries. In India the average age of heart disease is 42 years.

FREQUENTLY ASKED QUESTIONS

Q.   What is congestive heart failure?

A.   To a lay man it means sudden death. Medically it is failure of the heart to perform its functions – failure to cope with the demand of blood supply by body organs. In normal condition the heart is capable of coping with the demand of the body for actions like standing, walking and climbing. With the onset of the heart disease the capability of the heart goes on declining and heart may prove inadequate for mild physical activities. The patient is not able to perform normal functions without difficulty of breathing or stress. With further advancement in the impairment the patient becomes breathless and fatigued even at rest. In some cases, the heart stops functioning suddenly as in the case of acute coronary thrombosis or pulmonary edema. In other cases, like mitral valve disease and high blood pressure the breakdown of the heart's power is extremely slow and the process extends for months or years. In cases of aortic valve disease, in spite of severe valvular deformities the patient can lead normal life for years but may succumb to sudden failure of the heart.

Medical men can distinguish which part of the heart failed first. Most commonly the death in cardiac patients occurs due to left ventricular failure. Pumping action of the ventricles may be impaired due to many diseases. For example, the muscles of the heart may grow weak due to heart attack, infection or toxins (alcohol or chemotherapy agents). The apparent effect is on the ventricular contraction, also called systolic dysfunction. Disease such as Hemochromatosis (iron overload) or Amyloidosis* causes stiffening of the heart muscle and impaired capacity of the ventricle to relax and fill. This is known as diastolic dysfunction. Chronic high blood pressure also causes thickening of the heart wall. In hypothyroidism the oxygen demand of the body is increased and it may be difficult to supply blood to all the organs.

* Build-up of amyloid protein in the heart

In such a situation when the heart muscles are quite weak kidneys do not get enough blood which reduces the excretion of sodium as a result of which body retains more fluid. Lungs may be congested with fluid causing pulmonary edema and the patient experiences decreased ability to exercise. Similarly, liver and intestine are also affected. The hands and feet show edema.

Q.   What is myocardial infarction?

A.   Myocardial infarction (MI) or acute myocardial infection (AMI) is commonly known as heart attack. It results from the obstruction in the blood supply to part of the heart. In the coronary artery a plaque is formed which is an unstable collection of cholesterol and fatty acids, white bloods cells and fibrous tissue on the inner wall. This may take decades to build up. As a result of this growth, blood supply to a part of the heart is decreased and that part gets less oxygen and nutrients. The plaque may rupture and a part of it may completely occlude a smaller artery in few minutes. This leads to damage (myocardial infarction) to the supply area of that artery. This makes it difficult to supply blood & causes ischemia. The heart cells in the territory of the artery die. In that place a collagen scar is formed. This is a permanent damage to the heart muscle and the scar may lead the patient to life-threatening arrhythmias* and may result in the formation of ventricular aneurysm*[1] that may have severe effects.

Q.   What are the Signals of heart disease?

A.   The important signals of heart disease are:

I.   Excessive and increasing tiredness after day's work.

II.   Pain in arms and /or back and shoulders on working.

III.   Sweating and nausea.

IV.   Shortness of breath on exertion.

V.   Swelling of ankles or legs in the evening.

* Improper beating of the heart.
*[1] A large bulge & weakened area in an artery.

VI.   Pain in the chest behind the breast bone on climbing stairs or walking fast.

VII.   Scanty urine.

The doctor has to carefully examine the patient as some of these features occur in other diseases also. Shortness of breath is also found in anaemia, bronchial asthma and pneumonia while swelling on legs does occur in case of vitamin deficiency, anaemia and cirrhosis of liver. These symptoms have to be sorted out carefully. In diabetic patients some of these symptoms are not manifested and they may have a silent heart attack which is more dangerous as the patient does not get any time for treatment.

Some of the important symptoms during heart attack are as follows: -

•   Chest discomfort, which may feel like pain, pressure, tightness,

heaviness or burning.

•   Pain or discomfort in the neck, shoulders, lower jaw, arms, upper

back   or abdomen.
- Shortness of breath.
- Feeling lightheaded, dizzy or fainting.
- Nausea or vomiting.
- Unusual sweating.
- Fatigue.
- Heart palpitation, feeling heart beating fast or arrhythmic.

(8) Pain in chest

It is generally believed by people that the heart pain is on the left side of the body but pain in the centre of the chest is a prominent symptom of the heart trouble. True heart pain is mistaken as acidity or gas as a result of which the treatment is unnecessarily delayed. It is therefore said that a patient complaining of his stomach should be checked for heart and one complaining of heart should be checked for gastric problems. Sometimes the heart pain is replaced by hyperacidity or "heart burn" which is treated by antacid.

It should be remembered that any discomfort or pain in the centre of the chest after walking, climbing or on any other physical exertion associated with numbness in one or both arms should be taken as angina or cardiac pain. Although, it is alarming but this type of problem can be eased with simple measures like avoiding physical labor, reduction of body weight and having a positive approach. The patient should be treated rationally by friends and relatives otherwise he may develop into a "heart conscious person" and will act as invalid.

(9) Shortness of breath

In the early stages of the heart disease breathing difficulty is mild to the extent that it is hardly noticeable. Over the time the problem progressively worsens specially after walking and climbing. In the later stages the patient feels uncomfortable even when resting in the bed. In case of high blood pressure and coronary disease, a sudden attack of breathing difficulty may be experienced and the patient wakes up from the sleep. After an hour or two of discomfort the patient goes to sleep again when the discomfort subsides. This condition is known as cardiac asthma. Difficulty in respiration in heart disease exhibits typical pattern of deep breathing or sighing which interrupts normal breathing at irregular intervals.

(10) **Palpitation**

A normal person generally is not aware of his heart beat but when he becomes aware of thumping of the heart, it is known as palpitation. It depends on the sensitivity of the individual. A nervous or hypersensitive individual may be conscious of his heart beat after emotional excitement, physical effort or during convalescence from fever. Once disturbed he continues to feel his heart beat for a long time until examined by a doctor.

FREQUENTLY ASKED QUESTION

Q.   Why palpitation occurs?

Beating of the heart during palpitation may be regular or irregular. It may be slow, fast or very fast. When a specific part of the heart muscle becomes unduly irritable, the heart may produce extra beats from time to time disturbing the normal regular beating of the heart. In such a case the individual becomes conscious of his heart beat and leads to unnecessary alarm. These extra beats of the heart may be due to gas formation in the stomach or intestine, infected tooth or sinus or in heart disease.

(11) Sleep disturbances

Although it's not unusual to feel tired due to a lack of sleep or a particularly demanding week or month, you should take special notice of any unusual or prolonged disturbance in your sleep patterns. A recent study revealed that almost half of the women who had recently suffered a heart attack also experienced sleep disturbances in the days or weeks leading up to their attacks.

(12) Swelling

Swelling is in fact collection of fluids within the soft tissue of the body under the skin. This is reduced by administering diuretics (drugs that increase urine output). Swelling in both the ankles in the evening or on standing and walking for several hours is an important symptom for heart disease. It is absent in the morning hours. In the case of heart disease swelling is usually seen in the lowest part of the body, therefore, can be seen in the ankles and feet. In the patients who are confined to bed it appears near about the tail bone. Swelling in the cardiac patient is soft. On applying pressure by fingertip, a depression appears which persists for a few seconds.

(13) Pain in the arm

Numbness in the left arm is a symptom mostly associated with heart disease by lay man but it may be due to neuritis* or abnormality in the upper cervical region. Pain in the left arm generally appears on exertion and disappears after a few minutes. It is mostly associated with constriction in the chest. In case of coronary thrombosis pain appears in both the arms.

* Inflammation of nerve

(14) Fainting

Diseases of the heart have little to do with fainting; however, it may appear in the case of aortic valve disease or heart block. In a sensitive individual sudden emotional shock or change in posture may over stimulate the vagus nerve with sudden fall of blood pressure and slow beating of the heart, as a result of which the brain does not receive adequate amount of blood which leads to temporary loss of consciousness.

(16) HOCM

HOCM also known as hypertrophic cardiomyopathy is a disorder in which the muscle of the heart (myocardium) becomes thick due to unknown reason, which can be diagnosed by X-RAY. Despite enlargement in size the heart may supply sufficient blood to the body organs for a number of years. HOCM is known for causing surprise heart attack in any age group without showing any symptoms.

Sometime in cardiac patients the size of the heart increases which can be diagnosed by X-RAY. Complications like pneumonia, loss of blood, over exertion or pregnancy in such patients may lead to heart failure. In case of athletes the heart is usually enlarged this may cause problems in non-active post- retirement period.

FREQUENTLY ASKED QUESTIONS

Q. **Is heart disease more common in women?**

A. It was believed that only men have heart disease and women at risk only in older age. Recent studies show that about 1.3 million women have heart disease and their number increases every year. It is no more a disease of old age as 20% women under 65 have heart attack each year. Also, the rate of heart disease in men is declining but that in women is at rise. Still only 25% women recognize heart disease as a big cause of death world over. The British Heart Foundation highlighted in its report that only 12 % women are aware of the most important factors responsible for heart attack. The causes of heart ailment also show some differences from men. Type II diabetes increases the risk in women than in men. Women smokers are at higher risk than men. Depression is also a more important factor for heart disease in women than in men. Women taking contraceptive pills are a risk three times than in men. In some women blood pressure rises during pregnancy, but at the time of delivery it drops. Such women may have high blood pressure later in life.

Q. **Do women show different signs for heart attack?**

A study of National Institute of health (NIH) shows that women often experience new or different physical symptoms a month or more before experiencing heart attack. Among the 515 women studied 95% said they knew their symptoms were new or different quite before experiencing a heart attack. Women's symptoms are not as predictable as those of men.

Most women know the symptoms of a heart attack -- squeezing chest pain, shortness of breath and nausea. But as it turns out, these symptoms are more typical for males. Female heart attacks can be quite different -- and it's important for all women to learn the warning signs.

Rhonda Monroe's story is a cautionary tale. She was mystified when strong pain struck her left breast and left arm. Monroe, who was a 36-year-old mother of three, didn't know it at the time, but she was having early symptoms of a heart attack. "I certainly wasn't thinking about my heart because I was young and healthy and had been skinny," she says.

As the pain moved into her shoulder and back, Monroe took pain relievers. But the next day, she had nausea, sweating, vomiting, and chest pain. An ambulance rushed her to the emergency room.

Her next hurdle: getting the doctors to believe her. "They didn't take me seriously," Monroe says. She didn't fit the profile of a heart attack patient. The doctors told her she was too young, she was not overweight, and there was no family history of heart disease.

Frustrated by worsening pain and weakness Monroe returned to the hospital several times over the days that followed, only to come home with no answers.

Monroe turned to her primary care doctor about her situation and went through more tests at the hospital. Finally, she got her diagnosis -- a week after the initial breast and arm pain. As Monroe recalls, a cardiologist who had previously dismissed her complaints made the diagnosis. "The doctor told me, 'Well, it's a good thing you're persistent because you're having a heart attack.'"

Heart experts say Monroe's situation is all too common. Women who have "atypical" symptoms, such as arm or back pain or nausea, might not realize at first that they're having a heart attack.

Then when they do seek emergency care, doctors sometimes misdiagnose them.

**Q.	Is hormone replacement therapy useful for protecting the women from heart attack?**

A.	Till few years ago the doctors had been giving hormonal replacement therapy to menopausal women considering estrogen and progesterone as heart protector. But a 2002 US study showed that it did not protect the heart, rather it increased the risk of clotting. A trial of 17000 women was abandoned because many women developed breast cancer. Also, the rate of heart disease and stroke was also raised. It was suggested that they should take drug therapy and adopt dietary changes. However, women experiencing menopausal changes like hot flushes are still prescribed hormone replacement therapy.

**Q.	How does one know if her symptoms are serious?**

A.	It is better to make it a habit to note typical aches and pains and normal reactions to foods and activities. This may help in recognizing when something is wrong. If she has a risk factor like high blood pressure, high cholesterol, diabetes or sedentary lifestyle, she should be especially careful about monitoring how she feels or if she has any early signs of heart attack. If she feels worried or has unusual changes in her energy levels, comfort or sleep, she should discuss with the doctor.

Major symptoms prior to heart attack in women include:

- Unusual fatigue -70%
- Sleep disturbance—48%
- Shortness of breath—42%
- Indigestion—39%
- Anxiety—35%

Major symptoms during the heart attack include:

- Shortness of breath—58%
- Weakness in arms—55%

- Unusual fatigue—43%
- Cold sweat—39%
- Dizziness—39%

Some women may have heart attack without chest pain.

Q.   What is TIA?

A.   TIA, or transient ischemic attack, is a "mini stroke" that occurs when a blood clot blocks an artery for a short time. The only difference between a stroke and TIA is that with TIA the blockage is transient (temporary). TIA symptoms occur rapidly and last a relatively short time. Unlike a stroke, when a TIA is over, there's no permanent injury to the brain. There's no way to tell if symptoms of a stroke will lead to a TIA or a major stroke.

Q.   Is there any relation between heart disease and exercise in women?

A.   A study made on 74000 ethnically diverse post –menopausal women showed that those who walked for 30 minutes every day had lower risk of suffering a heart attack. Other studies have also confirmed this observation. It is therefore, very important to be physically active.

Q.   What is the relation between stress and heart disease?

A.   Level of stress varies from person to person. One may be under stress even if he has to do certain routine jobs like booking a railway ticket, bringing grocery and the like. A slight stress like being mindful of his duties is good as it helps increase your activity level. For other people stress with worry may be harmful. Some experts believe that stress affects the way the brain regulates the heart rate and can trigger irregular heartbeat. A stressful life induces people to drink, smoke and eat poorly and avoid exercise. It is therefore very important to adopt suitable methods to manage stress.

Q.   Is there any relationship between lycopene and heart disease in women?

A.   Lycopene is a constituent of tomato juice. It is helpful in many diseases. Study on ischemic heart risk factors shows that lower serum lycopene in women is associated with risk of heart attack and stroke. Dr Sesso has reported in the journal of nutrition that Women with high intake of lycopene rich tomato-based food had a reduced risk of cardiovascular disease as compared to women with low intake of these foods. Women having high level of lycopene (21.0 microgram /dl) also have high values of other beneficial carotenoids such as lutein, Zeaxanthin and alpha and beta carotene.

Q.   What should one do if he/she has symptoms of heart attack?

A.   If one knows that one has a heart problem, one must keep with them the phone number(s) of his cardiologist, the hospital which the cardiologist recommends and the ambulance.

- One must know the symptoms of heart attack. If one feels like having a heart attack, one should not wait. One should immediately call the doctor and the ambulance. One should not drive by themself to the hospital. Patients reaching the hospital by ambulance get early treatment than who reach by car, as paramedical in the ambulance begin treatment as soon as they reach the patients address.
- Should not try self-medication unless prescribed by the cardiologist.
- Chew and swallow one uncoated tablet of aspirin (325mg)
- The door should be open to let the emergency staff enter the room.
- Should sit in a comfortable chair while waiting

for help.
- Should keep phone at hand.
- Should not panic

Q.   How long do heart attack symptoms last?

**A.   **Knowledge of heart attack symptoms is very valuable for surviving a life-threatening heart attack. Every minute counts during heart attack. Fast action can save the life. Heart attack symptoms may be sudden and intense, but mostly start slowly and are mild. Appearance of heart attack symptoms varies from person to person. Symptoms may be present for days or even week before heart attack occurs. The symptoms may go away and come back.

Q.   What should I do when diagnosed with a heart problem?

A.   Coming to know news about having a heart problem leaves the patient and his family stunned with shock. They no longer remain in a position to discuss the disease with the doctor. One should not panic at such moments, rather should be calm. Try to take another appointment with the doctor after two- three days. That will give you time to do some research and find questions for future steps. At the second meeting, ask the doctor the questions and name of a specialist for second opinion. Many people skip this step. According to a recent survey, about 30 percent second opinion results in a different diagnosis and treatment. You shall get more accurate information and a specialized hand to treat.

Q.   What should I do if I see a man collapsing on the road?

A.   Many people die outside the hospitals on the road or in the market as they don't get immediate medical attention. One person was heading to station to catch a train. His heart stopped beating and he fell on the road, two bystanders rushed to him, one gave a call to the ambulance and the other performed CPR by pushing on the chest, the other tried mouth to mouth respiration. Within minutes the ambulance arrived and he was rushed to the hospital. He was unaware of three blockages in his arteries. He was lucky and recovered completely. Many are not so fortunate. According to Dr. Ian Stiell of the Ottawa Health Research Institute, "chances of survival are four times better if someone performs CPR on you, if you wait for the ambulance, it will be too late." It is a matter of great concern that people suffering heart attacks get immediate medical attention. Unfortunately, people make crowd around him doing nothing, rather obstructing others from doing something. It is important that more and more people are trained to help such patients. A lot many lives can be saved.

Q.   What is cardiac arrhythmia?

A.   Arrhythmias are the problems of the heart rhythm. Sometimes the heart pulse is extremely rapid, too slow, too early (premature contraction) or too irregular. This condition is apparent when electrical impulses are not working properly. Often people who experience atrial flutter might have hypertension, coronary artery disease or pathological changes in the myocardium. Sometimes atrial flutter may also be experienced without any known cause. Atrial flutter may go in short time but it may stay for months or years.

Many heart arrhythmias are harmless. Some arrhythmias when they deviate too much from the normal heart beat or take place in a weak or damaged heart may be troublesome or even fatal. When the heart rate is over 160 per minute or more, the condition is known as tachycardia. The condition is relatively harmless and subsides in minutes or hours without treatment. The resting heart rate sometimes goes below 60 beats per minute.

Mostly it is symptomatic at resting heart rate below 50 per minute. This condition is known as bradycardia. When the heart beat is irregular the arrhythmia is called fibrillation. When a single heart beat occurs before time it is known as premature contraction.

Q.   What causes cardiac arrhythmia?

A.   The electrical impulses that make the heart to contract follow a precise pathway to work properly. Any interruption to these impulses results in arrhythmia.

A drop in blood supply to the heart can alter the ability of the heart cells to conduct electric impulse. The spread of electrical impulses is affected if the heart has a dead or damaged tissue.

For a person with a healthy heart the process works properly, if the heart beat is between 60 and 100 beats per minute when resting. The lower the heart rate, fitter is the person. Olympic athletes usually have a resting heart rate less than 60 beats per minute because their hearts are very efficient. Professional cyclist Miguel Indurain had resting heart rate 28 beats per minute.

The cardiac defibrillator is a device which is used to terminate the potentially fatal arrhythmias. This device works by delivering an electric shock to the patient in order to regularize the function of a mass of muscle of the heart. This is known as "rebooting the heart". This therapy is time dependent and must be applied before the cardiopulmonary arrest.

Q.   What are the signs and symptoms of arrhythmia?

Some patients do not show any symptoms. The problem is detected usually during a routine medical checkup. Even if the patient notices a symptom, it does not necessarily mean that there is a serious concern. Sometimes the patients with life threatening arrhythmias may also not have any symptoms.

Symptoms of tachycardia are:

- Breathlessness
- Dizziness
- Syncopae (fainting or near fainting)
- Fluttering of the chest
- Lightheadedness
- Sudden weakness.

Sometimes there may be no symptoms.

Symptoms of bradycardia are:

- Angina
- Chest pain
- Difficulty when exercising
- Dizziness
- Fatigue
- Lightheadedness
- Syncopae
- Palpitations
- Shortness of breath

This may be due to the absence of electrical impulses from the sinoatrial node. generally fainting and shortness of breath is caused because those with bradycardia may not be pumping sufficient oxygen to their heart which affects the brain.

Resting bradycardia is often considered normal if the individual has no fatigue, dizziness, weakness, lightheadedness, fainting, chest pain, palpitation or shortness of breath associated with it. For infant's bradycardia is defined as a heart rate below 100 beats per minute (normal is around 120-160 beats per minute). Premature babies as compared to full term babies are likely to have apnea and bradycardia which is said to be due to under development of the centers in the brain that regulate breathing. Management of bradycardia depends whether or not the person is stable or unstable. If he is stable no emergent treatment is required. If he is unstable, he should be treated with atropine, dopamine or epinephrine.

Q.   What is constrictive pericarditis?

A. In this condition the outer covering of the heart (the pericardium) becomes inflamed. More commonly it is due to   some infection such as tuberculosis, however, it may due to heart attack or cardiac surgery.

Q.   Why does hypoglycemia cause tachycardia?

A.   When blood sugar is low, the adrenal glands are stimulated to release adrenalin, which is a quick acting hormone. It signals the liver and skeletal muscles to release glucose into the blood to keep the individual normal. Since adrenalin is a stress hormone, it also increases the heart, respiratory rate and vasoconstriction.

Q.   What is new for patients of cardiac arrhythmia?

A.   Wireless cardiac defibrillators are being implanted in patients. This device can monitor the cardiac rhythm and can start the heart if need be. Since this device is wireless the patient is no longer required to be hooked up to the machines during their check-up. Data transfer is easy which can be transferred by phone so the patient needs not to go to hospital so often for check-up.

Bundle Branch Block

As detailed earlier, our heart has a specialized conducting system through which the electrical impulse of contraction travels. This consists of S-A node (pace maker), A-V node and Bundle of His. The latter after its origin from the A-V node divides into right and left bundle branches which carry the electrical impulses to the respective ventricles. When any of the bundle branches is unable to conduct the impulse, it is known as bundle branch block. The chief effect of a bundle branch block is to disrupt the normal coordinated and simultaneous contraction of the two ventricles.

Right bundle branch block----- When blockage is in the right bundle branch the impulse does not travel through the right ventricle, therefore, theoretically there shall be no contraction in the right ventricle, but it receives delayed impulses from the left ventricle, so there is delayed contraction. In an electrocardiogram the QRS complex is wide. Adverse effects of right bundle branch depend upon the position of the block. If it is nearer the A-V node, it may have severe adverse effect. Normally with right bundle branch the individual can live for years.

Left bundle branch block--- It is rather more serious block because it hampers the rhythmic contraction of the left ventricle which has to pump the blood to all the body organs. Its severity also depends upon its position.

Q.   What are the symptoms of bundle branch block?

A.   If the heart of the individual has no other problem, he will not experience any discomfort with the block and may lead normal life for years. However, some people experience fainting (syncope) or like they are going to faint (presyncope). It may be a warning about a more serious heart ailment. It might indicate that a small part of your heart is not getting sufficient oxygenated blood. It has been found that those having left bundle branch have greater risk of heart disease than others.

There may also be partial block of the left bundle branch like "left anterior fascicular block" or "left posterior fascicular block". This indicates the block in any one of the branches of the left bundle branch.

Q.   How is bundle branch block diagnosed?

A. As first step of diagnosis the doctor takes an electrocardiogram which shows up the bundle branch block if present. It can also tell if the bundle branch block is left bundle branch or right bundle branch block. After this the doctor does echocardiography of the heart which reveals the site affected by the bundle branch block.

Q.   How is bundle branch block treated?

A.   Usually bundle branch block does not need a treatment, but patients who have other heart ailments require treatment. If bundle branch block is developed during a heart attack, then a pace maker is fitted to the patient, which regulates the rhythm of the heart after a heart attack.

To patients who have both bundle branch blocks along with increase in heart size and diseased heart muscle a new type of pacing known as cardiac resynchronization treatment (CRT) is given. This device co-ordinates the beating of the two ventricles by pacing them at the same time.

Q.   Is it necessary to go for a comprehensive cardiovascular check-up after angioplasty or bypass surgery?

A.   Yes, it is. Sometimes angiography fails even if stent has been placed in your artery. In bypass surgery also cases have been reported of reclogging of the arteries within six months. A thorough check-up will help your cardiologist to assess your general performance. If some parameter shows abnormal value, he may give you advice regarding exercise or change in medicine. This will give you enough confidence for better recoupment.

Q.   What is the life of a graft?

A.   The arterial graft has a life of about 15 years, if everything goes well which depends as to how well you follow the advice of your cardiologist, the exercise you take, the food you eat and the stress level you have, besides blood pressure and diabetes etc.

Q.   What is target heart rate and how it is calculated?

A.   You must know your Target Heart Rate (TRH). You get maximum benefit from your cardio vascular activity when you exercise in the zone of your target heart rate. In general, your TRH is 60-80% of your maximum heart rate. The Kervonen method of calculating THR is one of the most effective methods to determine target heart rate because it takes into account your resting heart rate. Follow the following steps:

1. First of all find your **resting heart rate** (RHR) by counting your pulse for one minute as soon as you wake up while still in the bed. Count it for consecutive three days. Suppose it is (62+65+63)/3 =63

2. Find your **maximum heart rate and heart rate reserve**

Subtract your age from 220. This is your maximum heart rate (HRmax). If you are 40 years old

220 - 40=180

3. Now subtract your RHR from HRmax. This gives you your HRmax Reserve

HRmax Reserve= 180 - 63=117

4. **Calculate the lower limit of your THR.**

To get 60% of the RHmax reserves multiplies by 0.6 and add your RHR to the answer:

(117 x 0.6) +63=133. Lower limit of your THR is 133.

5. **Calculate the upper limit of your THR**

To find out 80% of the HRmax reserve multiplies by 0.8 and adds your RHR to the answer:

$(117 \times 0.8) + 63 = 157$

6. Combine the values obtained in steps 4 and 5 and divide by 2

Target Heart Rate TRH= $(133+157) / 2 = 145$. You can get the same result by simply multiplying HRmax reserve by 0.07 and adding it to RHR.

Q.   Can defects in fetal heart be detected?

A.   With the help of ultra sound major defects in the fetal heart can be detected, like transposition of the great arteries, hypoplastic left ventricular syndrome, atrioventricular septal defects, coarctation of the aorta and large ventricular septal defects.

Q.   How to have heart healthy life with diabetes?

A.   People with diabetes having high blood glucose level over a long period may have damage in the lining of the blood vessels. This causes roughness and makes it prone to clot formation. It is necessary to have regular check-up of blood glucose level and adopt a life style to keep blood glucose controlled with proper food and exercise.

Q.   How are emotions related with heart?

A.   According to the folk wisdom, the heart is the seat of intuition, love, creativity, gratitude faith and the like. How do we know this? We know it in our heart. There is no clear scientific basis for this remark, however new researches may lead to a definite role of emotions on the heart. It is found that heart produces certain hormones which balance other hormones. It is claimed that love hormone oxytocin, the hormone which is in action when mother feeds and tends her child is also produced by the heart. If it comes true, it may be possible to explore the mystery of heart's role in emotions. Also, there are many neurotransmitters working between heart and brain. There is some evidence that anxiety may be involved in triggering myocardial infarct. Acute anxiety may lead to hyperventilation which may cause vasospasm. It has also been suggested that there is acute effect of emotion on parameters like platelet aggregation and risk of thrombosis. Anger increases circulating levels of adrenalin which may induce inflammation in blood vessels. A good deal of research suggests that depression has a strong role in coronary deaths and myocardial infarcts.

Q.   Are there any agencies which provide funds for heart operation?

A.   There are some agencies which provide financial help to heart patients, mostly to young children. An organization "Save a Child" through teams from youth groups, schools, colleges and church is actively engaged in this activity. They claim to save a child's life every 29 minutes. Chief Minister Fund in all the states of India also provides fund for treatment. Organizations like Lions club and others may be approached. An internet search may provide more information.

Q.   Is sex safe for heart disease patient?

A.   According to the American Heart Association, it is probably safe to have sex if your cardiovascular disease has stabilized. It is better to consult your doctor before you resume sexual activity. Don't skip medication that could improve cardiovascular symptoms because they could impact your sex drive or function. If you are a woman and planning to be pregnant or starting birth control, be sure to talk to your doctor. If you are postmenopausal women with cardiovascular disease, it is safe to use estrogen vaginally inserted for treatment of painful intercourse.

Drugs to treat erectile dysfunction are generally safe, but it is safer not to use them if you are taking nitrate therapy for chest pain due to coronary artery disease.

Q.   Is sex life affected with heart disease?

A.   Many cardiovascular diseases especially hypertension and peripheral vascular disease cause changes in small blood vessels supplying blood to the legs, feet and genitals. When penis or vagina does not get proper supply of blood, there is impact on the arousal and engagement in sexual activity. Erectile dysfunction in 30-50% in males is due to blood vessel disease. Additionally, fatigue, shortness of breath, chest pain and general weakness which are associated with cardiovascular diseases may be responsible for sexual dysfunction. In some patients there may be fear that sexual activity may cause heart attack. This may also be a factor to decrease sexual function. Some medicines used for treatment of hypertension may also have negative side effects on sexual desire or erectile dysfunction.

Q.   Can these sexual disorders be reversed?

A.   In many cases individuals with cardiovascular disease may resume sexual activity and can be treated for sexual dysfunction if they strictly follow the doctor's recommendations and treatment plan. Bringing some life style changes like quitting smoking, avoiding alcohol consumption and regular physical activity and exercise can improve blood flow and the sexual dysfunction.

Q.   What happens immediately after bypass surgery?

A.   After bypass surgery you are taken to recovery room or directly to the intensive care unit (ICU) and kept on automatic ventilator with a thick tube thrust into your wind pipe. You are connected to monitors that display your ECG, blood pressure readings, breathing rate and oxygen level. When you come in sense, the nurse disconnects you from the ventilator, and puts you on a manual ventilator with a rubber bulb. You are asked to constantly press the bulb to throw air in to your lungs. When tired you stop pressing the bulb and the ventilator gives an alarm. The nurse rushes to you and asks you to keep pressing the bulb. After some time when you resume normal respiration and have stabilized, the tube from the wind pipe is removed. Here you feel some difficulty perhaps due to anesthesia induced weakness and tube in the wind pipe you are unable to speak. You feel your voice is almost gone. After some time, you gain a hoarse and weak voice, which takes about two days to be normal. Even after you start respiring normally, still you remain in a state of confusion and you sleep most of the time. The nurse assists you in coughing every two hours. Here you may find problem due to hoarseness, but it is necessary to keep removing mucous from collecting in the lungs. Hugging tightly a pillow against your chest will ease the discomfort. When you want to urinate, the nurse does not provide you the urine pot, instead takes you to the lavatory walking on your feet. It is to give your legs movement, as they did not work for some time, otherwise they will take longer time to achieve normal movement. After one day you are shifted to another ICU, if your progress is satisfactory. Time to time you are given an apparatus for exercise of lungs. As you improve and your condition stabilizes your IV drip is reduced or removed as per the condition. You are now given liquid diet. Your diet may be advanced to more solid food as you are able to tolerate them. Next day you are shifted to the ward. You are asked to walk 3-4 times each day. You may be required to stay in the hospital for a week or so.

Q. **What care should be taken at home after operation?**

A. Keep the surgical area clean and dry. Take bath as per the instructions given at the hospital. Do not drive until doctor allows. Talk to the doctor if you have fever or/ and chills, redness, swelling or bleeding or other drainage at the site of incision.

DIAGNOSTIC TOOLS

1.   **Electrocardiography (ECG)**

When a patient complains of chest pain, the doctor first tries to record an ECG. It is a device to interpret the electrical activity of the heart over a period of time, detected by the help of the electrodes attached to the skin. ECG is performed for diagnostic or research purpose on human beings and on experimental animals. It measures the rate and regularity of the heart beats, as well as the size and position of the chambers, any damage to the heart and the effect of drugs on the heart. In a myocardial infarction (MI) the ECG can identify if the heart muscle has been damaged in a specific area. This device cannot measure the pumping ability of the heart for which other tests like echocardiography and nuclear medicine tests are performed.

A typical ECG tracing of the heart activity shows a P wave, a QRS complex, a T wave and a U wave (which is not seen in all ECG recordings). The baseline voltage of ECG is known as isoelectric line which is measured as the segment of the tracing prior to P wave and following the T wave. The T wave represents the recovery of the ventricle. If in an ECG the T wave shows downward progression, it represents an ischemic heart that means the heart is not getting adequate amount of oxygen.

This test may be helpful for people with fainting, irregular heart rate and family history of heart disease. It is also used for screening of athletes for risk of sudden death and for those having high blood pressure to find abnormal thickening of the heart muscle.

2.   **Tread mill Test**

This test is used to study the ECG during stress. The person is subjected to walk on the moving strap at definite speed. The speed is increased gradually till heart rate become quite high. The doctor monitors hear rate and blood pressure. Immediately after walking, recovery period is also recorded. This test is useful for the people who are sedentary, having pain in chest, arm, neck or back and have shortness of breath.

3.   Echocardiography

Now a days echocardiography is being used as a routine method as a diagnostic tool for cardiac ailments because it is non-invasive, highly accurate and has no known risks and side effects. In transthoracic echocardiography (Heart ultrasound) the probe is placed on the chest wall of the subject and images are taken on a computer for studying and recording.

This test provides information about the size and shape of the heart chambers, presence and location of any damaged muscle. It may be obtained along with Doppler evaluation giving clear picture about the valves for any abnormality in them and about any back flow of blood due to valvular defect. Echocardiography can detect any abnormality in the motion of the heart wall which tells about insufficient supply of blood to that part of the heart (ischemia) which may be associated with coronary artery disease. Beside this echocardiography can detect any pathological changes in the heart muscle and can assess pumping efficiency of the heart.

4.   Transesophageal echocardiography

This technique is utilized when the images obtained by thoracic echocardiogram are not clear. In this case the probe is passed in to the subject's esophagus so that clear images may be obtained along with Doppler evaluation.

5. Stress Echocardiography

This method uses ultrasound images to assess the motion of the heart wall in response to the exercise (stress). Initially images are taken at resting heart rate to obtain base line data and then the subject is asked to walk on the tread mill to increase the heart rate up to 80% of the target heart rate (target heart rate = 220 (-) age of the subject). Then the images of the heart are taken at stress. If there is any abnormality in the wall motion it indicates coronary artery disease which has to be ascertained by angiography.

6. Three-dimensional echocardiography

This technique uses an ultrasound probe, some transducers and a processing system. This system provides images of a number of virtual slices of the heart in many planes which are reconstructed into a three-dimensional echocardiogram of the heart which helps in understanding any congenital malformations of the heart. It also helps in taking biopsies.

7. Contrast echocardiography

It is helpful in assessing the left ventricular endocardial margins, left ventricular volume and ejection fraction. With this technique better visualization of the wall thickening, structural abnormalities and myocardial ischemia may be made.

8. Coronary angiography

This technique is widely used in heart patients to ascertain the blockages in the coronary arteries. This involves cardiac catheterization i.e., to insert a device into a blood vessel to reach the heart. First of all, a local anesthesia is injected into the skin to make the area numb. Then a puncture is made in the femoral artery in the groin region or in the radial artery in the wrist. Subsequently a guide wire is pushed in to the artery. A plastic sheath which has a stiff plastic introducer inside it is then threaded over the wire and pushed into the artery. This catheter assembly is moved towards the heart and on reaching the aortic valve, the guide wire is removed. The catheter is then put at the opening of the origin of the coronary artery (either left or right) and x-ray opaque iodine-based contrast material is injected. The contrast material in the blood absorbs x-rays and gives fluorescent imaging by way of which the condition of the artery is visualized. If there are any plaques or blockage the lumen of the artery looks narrow or devoid of any blood. The image is taken at 2 to 3 frames per second on film or a CD. When the necessary procedure is complete, the catheter is removed. The site of insertion is firmly pressed to prevent bleeding.

Once the catheter is in place, it can be used to perform a number of procedures angioplasty and balloon septostomy.

9. Computed tomography angiography (CTA)

It is a non-invasive procedure to find out the condition of blood vessels in any area of the body. It is less costly. There is less discomfort as mostly thorax is subjected to investigation. This technique combines the use of x-rays with computerized analysis of the images. Beams of x-rays are passed from a rotating device through the area of interest from several angles and projection images are obtained, which are converted by the computer into three-dimensional picture of the area.

This technique is useful in screening for arterial disease because it displays the anatomical details more precisely than MRI or conventional catheter angiography. CTA is safer and much less time consuming than catheter angiography as the contrast material is injected in the arm vein and not in the large artery in the groin region. CTA is also used to identify arterio-venous malformations and in dissection in the aorta in which case the layers of the artery wall peel off from each other as a result of which the patient feels pain and it may be life threatening.

CTA involves certain risks also but care should be taken in case of the complications if any. There is a risk of allergic reaction when contrast material containing iodine is injected. A patient sensitive to x-ray dye is given special medication for 24 hours prior to CTA. It should be avoided in patients with kidney disease or severe diabetes because x-ray contrast material may further damage the kidneys. CTA may also increase life time cancer risk. However, there are many conditions when CTA is much useful and outweighs the risks which can be taken care of. One should keep a record of X-rays and CT scans and other radiation tests and alert the doctor, if he suggests any such test that you have already gone.

10. CARDIAC CT FOR CORONARY CALCIUM SCORING

It is a simple and convenient test for identification for coronary artery disease (CAD). It is CT Angiography as described earlier. It looks for calcium in the wall of the arteries. The amount of calcium found in the artery tells about the risk of a heart disease. It helps the doctor to give appropriate treatment for slowing the progress of coronary artery disease. This procedure does not need injection of contrast material and is completed in 15 minutes. Those having high cholesterol level, diabetes, a family history of heart disease, high blood pressure, smoking habit, inactive life and are obese should take this test.

Calcium score predicts the coronary artery disease as follows:

Calcium score	Presence of CAD
0	No evidence of CAD
1-10	Minimum evidence of CAD
11-100	Mild evidence of CAD

| 101-400 | Moderate evidence of CAD |
| Over 400 | Extensive evidences of CAD |

This test is good for people of age more than 50 years. In people less than 50 years calcium score may be low but they may have CAD.

ATRIAL SEPTAL DEFECT (ASD)

Arial septum is the partition wall between the two atria or the upper chambers of the heart. Septal defects are sometimes called a "hole" in the heart. In the fetal heart an opening known as foramen Ovale is present, but it closes before birth. After birth, the opening is no longer needed and usually closes or becomes very small within several weeks or months. Sometimes this opening does not close and remains large after birth. As many as one in five healthy adults still have a small leftover opening in the wall between the atria, called a Patent Foramen Ovale (PFO). The cause of this is not known, but it is believed to be a genetic manifestation. If the hole is quite small there is very little effect on the heart. When a large hole remains in the atrial septum, a large amount of oxygen-rich (red) blood leaks from the heart's left side back to the right side. Then this blood is pumped back to the lungs, despite already having been refreshed with oxygen. This causes heart to work more. Due to extra amount of blood, the pulmonary arteries are also damaged. Those having large opening in the atrial septum suffer with mild shortness of breath with exercise. The increased blood in the lung may increase patient's susceptibility to bronchial asthma. With progressive damage to the lung vessels, the pressure in the lung may rise, and the patient may suffer with Eisenmenger's syndrome. Such defects may be corrected in early childhood. In case of small hole, the patient need not to go under surgery, however if the hole is large, it is closed either by catheterization or by open heart surgery. Even when the defect is discovered in adulthood, patients benefit from closure of the large hole.

People with small unrepaired or repaired atrial septal defects rarely have any late problems. Those who have palpitations or who faint need to be evaluated by their cardiologist and may need medical therapy. Also, if the ASD is diagnosed late in life, the heart's ability to pump may have been affected, leading to heart failure. This condition requires treatment with diuretics to improve the pumping of the heart and to control blood pressure.

MAJOR RISK FACTORS

1.   High Blood Pressure or hypertension

When blood is pumped from the heart into the blood vessels, it exerts certain pressure on the wall of the blood vessels. This is known as blood pressure. It varies in different blood vessels and is highest in the blood vessels nearest the left ventricle which is the chamber of the heart from where the blood is pumped to the body organs. In modern life style where people are subjected to continuous stress to meet the daily needs, anxiety of paying mounting taxation and increasing cost of children's education, all together reflect upon the health of the people initiating with hypertension

Q.   What are the symptoms of high blood pressure?

A.   High blood pressure, if not quite high,generally shows no symptoms. Mostly people come to know about hypertension only when their blood pressure is checked by a doctor. People who have markedly elevated blood pressure may show the following symptoms :

Headache
Dizziness
Blurred vision
Nausia and vomiting
Chest pain and shortness of breath
Frequent urination
Nervous tension and
Fatigue

Q.   What is normal blood pressure?

A.   Blood pressure (BP) reading is recorded as systolic / diastolic. Systolic blood pressure means the blood pressure when the heart contracts while diastolic blood pressure is the blood pressure when the heart relaxes.

Normal BP: Less than 120/80 mm/hg

Prehypertension BP: 120~130/80~90 mm/hg

Stage 1 high blood pressure : 140~159/90~99 mm/hg

Stage 2 high blood pressure: 160 mm/hg and above/100 mm/hg and above

Q, What causes high blood pressure?

A   High blood pressue is not caused due to any specific factor but following factors may play important role in its development:

- Smoking. Nicotine increases the resting heart rate and increases the release of adrenaline that tends to increase blood pressure.
- Being over weight or obese.
- Lack of physical activity.
- Too much salt intake.
- Too much alcohol consumption.
- Hectic life style and Stress.
- Older age.
- Hardening of arteries.
- Genetics.
- Family history of high blood pressure.
- Chronic kidney disease.
- Adrenal and thyroid disorders.
- Other metabolic disorders.
- Habit of taking fast food.

In 15 % cases of hypertension the causative factors may be a damaged kidney, enlarged prostate, tumour of the brain, suprarenal or pituitary gland or overactive thyroid. This is known as secondary hypertension which becomes normal once the disease is cured .

Depending on the rate of progression of the disease hypertension has been differentiated into two types.

1.　　　Essential hypertension—This type accounts for 90% of cases. Causative factor remains obscure. Esssential blood pressure is greatly influenced by the diet and life style.It progresses slowly and the patient can lead a normal life for years. Salt intake is quite important factor. People living on the northern island of Japan eat more salt than any one in the world and have highest incidence of essential hypertension. People who add no salt to their diet have no incidence of hypertension.Majority of hypertension patients are salt sensitive. If they take salt more than the required, there is increase in blood pressure.

2.　　　Secondary hypertension—The disease is rapidly progressive which may be due to failure of kidneys. The blood pressure may exceed 300mm/Hg systolic and 150mm/Hg diastolic. Birth control pills those containing oestrogen as well as pregnancy may boost blood pressure as do the medicines that constrict blood vessels.

It is now known that the hypertension is accomplished with the narrowing of the arterioles. Beside this, increase in blood volume, thickening of blood, loss of elasticity of large vessels and powerful pumping action of the heart may be responsible for rise in blood pressure. The side -effects of hypertension largely depend on the duration of the disease and damage to the blood vessels rather than the height of blood pressure. When blood supply to vital organs is defective many complications may arise like angina pectoris, coronary thrombosis, heart failure, cardiac asthma, stroke or impaired vision. However,early treatment of hypertension may ward off any such complications.

Specific dietetic regimes are recommended for hypertensive patients who exclude fats, salt, protein and calories, but it does not always work because the patient does not accept the taste and does not take full diet leading to weakness and neurosis. Restricted diet may be necessary if the patient shows tendency of obesity and excessive retention of water or has a badly strained heart.

Q.   How does alcohol affect the heart?

A.   When alcohol is consumed it is absorbed into the blood stream, and affects the brain and the spinal cord, which are responsible for controlling virtually all body functions. Contrary to the popular belief alcohol is a depressant that slows down the functions of the nervous system. It affects emotions, hearing, movement, perception and vision. Taken in small amount alcohol can make the drinker less anxious and relaxed. Recent studies have shown that even modest amounts of alcohol consumption can cause blood pressure, especially in old people. When the quantity consumed is large, it causes more severe effects including confusion and disorientation. Long term drinking can increase the stress hormone cortisol which contracts blood vessels. When blood vessels supplying blood to the heart muscle are contracted, the heart muscle is starved of oxygen and nutrition and dies, causing heart attack. The risk of atrial fibrillation, the irregular heart beat can lead to stroke. Risk of stroke increases within the first few hours after heavy drinking. Withdrawal from alcohol consumption also causes health implications like sleep disruption, diabetes and mood disturbances, which are responsible for heart ailment.

Q.   What are the consequences associated with stage 2 hypertension?

A.   Some of the initial consequences of untreated hypertension are:

- Damage of kidney cells which may lead to kidney failure
- Damage of the retina which may lead to impaired vision
- Damage of arterial wall
- Stroke
- Heart attack
- Heart failure and death.

Q.   How is blood pressure measured?

A.   Normally for convenience the blood pressure is measured in the brachial artery in the arm with the help of an instrument known as sphygmomanometer in which the reading is made on the mercury scale. For measuring blood pressure of a person, the blood pressure cuff containing the deflated rubber bag is wound around the arm above the elbow.The bag is then inflated with the help of a rubber bulb, until the pulse on the wrist is no longer felt. With the help of the screw air from the bladder is slowly released.The point at which the pulse reappears is known as the systolic pressure.

For recording both systolic and diastolic blood pressure the ausculatory method is used. In this case also the cuff containing the deflated rubber bag is wound around the arm above elbow and the bag is inflated. The chest piece of the stethoscope is placed firmly on the artery at the angle of elbow, and the sounds are heared as gradual deflation of the rubber bag takes place. The point at which the first clear sound is heared is recorded as systolic pressure. Then the bag is deflated and the point at which the arterial sound disappears, is recorded as the diastolic blood pressure.

     Electronic blood pressure instruments are now available.You have to wear it on the left wrist, keeping the hand at the level of the heart and start it as per instructions. Soon it measures blood pressure and pulse rate.

If there is a difference of more than 15 mm/Hg between the systolic pressure of both the arms, it represents a dialated aorta or aortic aneurism. If the blood pressure of the arm is higher than that of the leg it suggests a type of congenital disease. If the blood pressure in the leg is more than that of thr arm, it indicates leakage in the aortic valve.

Blood pressure in nervous individuals at a medical examination is generally high because it is influenced by the physical, mental and emotional factors. Otherwise, they have normal blood pressure. This is known as White coat (office) hypertension.

Q.   What measures should be taken to treat hypertension?

A.   It is better to have a healthy life style to treat or prevent hypertension.   Some of the following suggestions may be useful: -

- Lose weight, if obese or over weight.
- Quit smoking.
- Eat healthy diet (more fruits and vegetables and less fat and dairy products
    and saturated fats).
- Eat less salt (not more than 2.00g /day).
- Take regular exercise for 30 minutes a day. Regular Exercise helps to
    eliminate body fat, lowers total cholesterol and raises HDL cholesterol that
    prevents fatty - cholesterol deposits.
- Limit alcohol drinks to two drinks a day for men and one drink a day for
    women.

Q.   What types of drugs are recommended for hyperten-

sion?

A. There are several types of drugs used to treat hypertension

- Angiotensin converting enzyme inhibitors.
- Angiotensin II receptor blockers.
- Alpha blockers.
- Alpha agonists.
- Renin inhibitors.
- Combination medications.

As the first line of therapy diuretics are given to most people having hypertension.

Besides the above, reserpine an alkaloid of plant *Rauwolfia serpentina* is also found very effective. No drugs should be taken without doctor's advice.

Generic and brand names and side effects of the medicines being taken must be known. While travelling one should keep all the drugs with him or her. Drugs should not be changed without asking the doctor.

Q.   Does high blood pressure prevent from sex?

A. During sexual activity blood pressure and heart rate increases even in a normal person. It is reported that at the climax of sex the heart rate almost doubles in a normal person. Respiration rate and blood pressure also increase. With these observations the general belief is that those having high blood pressure should abstain from sex. But it is not the correct conclusion. One of the consequences of high blood pressure is weakening of the heart, which results in insufficient blood supply from the heart to various parts of the body. Improper blood supply also causes erectile dysfunction. Doctors suggest that not the sex but the strenuous sex is bad for the heart. Following points may be helpful in having sex with high blood pressure: -

1. Stomach should not be full—after a meal more blood flows towards digestive system. If the heart is weak, it may not bear

strenuous sexual activity.

2. Alcohol—excessive alcohol consumption increases heart rate, so the heart is already under extra workload. It is, therefore, recommended that those having a weak heart should not indulge in sex after too much alcohol intake.

3. Fatigue- A tired person should avoid sex, should rather go to sleep.

4. Stress—if there is a sense of guilt or fear of illicit sex, it may be harmful for a person with a weak heart.

If a person experiences chest pain during sex and it persists even after sex, it should be taken as heart pain, which shows that the heart has been put to stress. If high pulse rate and breathlessness continue for fifteen minutes after sex, a doctor should be approached. Persons having high blood pressure can have normal sex, if they are regularly taking drugs to control blood pressure.

Q.   What is Ayurvedic approach to hypertension?

A.   Ayurveda often called science of life is a very old science, which has been practiced in India since ancient times. The medical fraternity has now agreed that India's ancient stream of medicine has some miracle cures for cardio-vascular diseases. This science is based on the principle that the patient should be treated as a whole and not only is his disease treated. According to Ayurveda disease is caused when there is imbalance of all the doshas (Pitta, vata and kapha). Of these the most important is vata as it controls the other two doshas-Pitta and Kapha. If any of these doshas increases excessively high, it results in ailment. A skilled Ayurvedic practitioner can diagnose the ailment by feeling the pulse of the patient. In Ayurveda, hypertension is known as *"Raktavata"*. It involves heart and blood vessels. People with pitta and vata constitution are more prone to hypertension. Anger, frustration, irritability, anxiety and fear lead to mal-functioning of endocrine glands leading to hypertension. In the treatment of hypertension emphasis is given on nutrition, exercise (pranayama), yoga, meditation, behavioral modifications along with various herbs and minerals. Ayurveda also recommends weight loss, regular exercise and taking low fat diet as described elaborately in *"Medoroga Chikitsa"*. Ethical elements for improving life style are described in "Achara *Rasayan"*. Love and affection can immensely help in lowering blood pressure. Telling lies, speaking loudly and getting annoyed during conversation may increase blood pressure. Laughter is good relaxation therapy, which should be used to overcome stress. For complete tranquility of mind, one should meditate in the "shava *Asan"* first concentrating on the incoming and outgoing breath for about ten minutes. By practicing regularly, mental disturb-. ance diminishes and blood pressure minimizes. Then meditate. Chanting the mantra "OM" or listening recording of it in the early morning or evening is also beneficial

Some plant preparations are also recommended:

1.   Sarpgandha – For centuries,*Rauwolfia sepentina* has been used to treat hypertension.

2.   Arjuna—*Terminalia arjuna* induces dose dependent hypotension. It has liver protecting and cardio protecting, hypolipidemic, antianginal and has anti-atheroma properties.

3.   Gokshura—*Tribulus terrestris* is used in treating many diseases including hypertension. It is diuretic and acts as ACE inhibitor.

4 Punarvava— *Boerhaavia diffusa* is diuretic and has Ca_2^+ channel blocking activity.

According to the dosha predominance in hypertension following may be used:

When vata predominates, there is increase in blood pressure along with insomnia and anxiety. The Ayurvedic practitioners recommend

(1)   Taking a 125mg mixture of serpgandha and jatamansi for

2-3 months.

(2)   One clove of garlic with honey one or two times a week.

(3)   Taking saraswat and nutmeg powder in warm milk.

(4)   Taking ashwgandha preparations.

When pitta predominates, the patient suffers from irritability, anger, violent headaches and sensitivity to light along with varying blood pressure. Some people also suffer from nose bleeding. Recommended treatment includes drugs having cold potency:

(1)   Taking 250mg of Brahmi at night regularly for a month

(2)   Taking Brahmirasayan

(3)   Taking saraswat powder

(4)   Taking 1gram of Indian sarsaparilla(sariva) for 15 days

When Kapha predominates, there may be dull headache, oedema, and lethargy. Blood pressure remains continuously high. Treatment recommends the use of gugglu, cardamom and cinnamon.

Garlic is also credited to decrease triglycerides level in the blood by about 10 percent, thus lowering blood pressure.

Cow urine therapy is also said to be helpful in hypertension.

It is claimed to have anti-inflammatory, antioxidant, stress reducing, antihypertensive and diuretic properties. Some people also take small about, half cup of self-urine every morning for better health and hypertension.

2.   Cholesterol

Cholesterol is a fatty chemical compound that is synthesized in our body and is found in all cell membranes, skin cells, nerve cells, heart cells, arteries, veins just a few to name. It is utilized in the formation of cell membrane and certain hormones like estrogen, progesterone and testosterone, bile to absorb fat soluble vitamins A, D, E, and K and is a precursor to endogenous vitamin D production. Liver is the chief producer of cholesterol while some part of it comes from our diet. Dietary sources of cholesterol are meat, poultry, fish and dairy products. Foods of plant origin contain no cholesterol.

FREQUENTLY ASKED QUESTIONS

Q. **What are Triglycerides?**

A. They are another form of fat which provide energy, and help in formation of cell membrane. Their each molecule consists of one molecule of glycerol and three molecules of fatty acids. They are largely present in meat, dairy products and cooking oils. Triglycerides are also synthesized by liver from fats and sugars. The term fats or lipids include both cholesterol and triglycerides. Since these fats do not mix well with blood, so they attach to blood protein and are then known as lipoproteins particles. They reach through blood to various parts of the body to be utilized.

There are three main types of lipoprotein particles.

1. Low density lipoproteins (LDL) about 2/3 part of total blood cholesterol are
    LDL.
2. High density lipoproteins (HDL)

3. Very low-density lipoproteins (VLDL). Fats synthesized by the liver are
    transported to the blood in the form of VLDL.
4. In addition to these, there are chylomicrons, often they attach to the fats
    received from food and carry it to liver and fat deposition sites.

Q. **What are good and bad lipoprotein particles?**

A. LDL is Low density lipoprotein and is known as bad cholesterol because it is associated with an increased risk of heart disease, stroke and peripheral artery disease. LDL lipoprotein circulates through the body with the blood and deposits cholesterol on the inner wall of the artery, causing formation of the cholesterol plaque. Over the time the wall of the artery thickens and the plaque narrows the cavity of the artery, as a result of which less blood flows through by the artery. This condition is known as atherosclerosis. HDL (high density lipoprotein) is good cholesterol because they interfere with the accumulation of LDL cholesterol in the artery wall and   prevent atherosclerosis by   sending it to the liver to be disposed off. High LDL and low HDL levels are risk factors. In some families very low or very high HDL levels may be found. Families with low HDL cholesterol level have a higher incidence of heart attack than the others, while families with high HDL cholesterol levels live longer with a lower frequency of heart attack. HDL level is found low in persons who smoke, are overweight and are inactive, and in people with type II diabetes mellitus. It is high in people who do not smoke, are lean and exercise regularly.

Q.   **What are animal and vegetable fats?**

A.   Fats obtained from animal sources have more saturated fatty acids (SFA). They solidify on cooling and are undesirable for heart health as they help in enhancing the blood cholesterol. If more in amount they decrease the potential of liver for removing LDL from circulation. Fish oil fats are different as they have low saturated fat and cholesterol. They have many varieties of unsaturated fat known as Omega 3 polyunsaturated fatty acids (Omega 3 PUFA). They have beneficial effect as they reduce blood triglyceride levels and lower the risk of blood clotting.

Q.   **What is the fate of dietary cholesterol and triglycerides?**

A.   Dietary fats after digestion in the intestine are absorbed by the blood and taken to liver and fat deposit sites like muscles, abdomen and below the waist. VLDL carries triglycerides to body tissues to be utilized for energy production. After this VLDL converts into LDL which is rich in cholesterol. If inflamed sites are found, the LDL cholesterol deposits cholesterol there. It may be deposited on the inner wall of the arteries. Prolonged deposits may form plaque. With the breakdown of the tissues free cholesterol is generated. HDL takes this cholesterol from the blood and from the plaque site to the liver for being recycled or for the formation of bile.

**Q.	What is safe cholesterol level?**
A.	National Institute of Health recommends that the cholesterol of a person should be maintained under 200 mg/dl. Its level from 200 to 239 mg/dl is considered as borderline high. Levels from 240mg/dl and above are considered as high.

**Q.	Is HDL more in women high?**
A.	In women desirable HDL level is 55 mg/dl as compared to man (45 mg/dl) because of estrogen.

**Q.	What are desirable levels of LDL, VLDL and triglycerides?**
A.	Optimum LDL should be between 100-129mg/dl. From 130 to 159 is considered as borderline high while 160 to 189mg/dl is high and above 190mg/dl is very high. Those having heart disease should maintain LDL level below 100mg/dl.
VLDL should be less than 28mg/dl. Optimum Triglyceride level is less than 150mg/dl. From 150 -199mg /dl is borderline high. From 200 – 499 mg/dl is high and above 500mg/dl is very high.

**Q.	What are the factors that matter most for abnormal lipid profile?**
A.	Factors that affect blood cholesterol levels include oily diet, age, diabetes, hypothyroidism, heredity, unhealthy life style and medical disorders.	High triglyceride level may be due to increased formation of triglycerides by liver, less storage at deposition sites, conversion of sugar in to triglycerides, excessive dietary sugar, fat and alcohol. Disorders like diabetes, kid-

ney disease and obesity also increase triglyceride level.

Q.   What may cause low HDL cholesterol level?
A.   There is inverse relationship between HDL and triglycerides. If triglycerides are high, HDL level will be low. In some people it is a genetic manifestation. Excessive intake of PUFA rich oil and less physical activity induces low HDL level. Other factors include diabetes mellitus, tobacco chewing, and smoking and excessive weight gain. Use of oral contraceptive pills also reduces HDL level and increase cholesterol.

Q.   How often cholesterol level should be checked?
A.   As per National Institute of Health guidelines cholesterol level should be checked every five years after 20. If elevated levels are found, tests should be made more frequently.

Q.   What is total cholesterol/HDL ratio?
A.   The total cholesterol to HDL cholesterol ratio is the number used to determine the risk of developing atherosclerosis. 3.3-4.4 is low risk; 4.5-7.0 is average risk. 7.0 -11.0 is moderate risk, while more than 11.0 is high risk.

Q.   What is LDL/HDL ratio?
A.   Desirable ratio is 0.5-3.0, 3.1 – 6.1 is moderate risk and above 6.0 is high risk. One percent increases in HDL cuts your risk of heart disease by 2 to 3 percent.

Q.   What are the drugs useful in lowering cholesterol level?
A.   Drugs available for lowering cholesterol level include statins, bile acid resins, and fibric acid derivatives. These drugs are most effective when they are taken with low cholesterol, trans-fat and saturated fat diet. Doctor must be consulted before taking cholesterol lowering drugs. All the brands of statin are not effective for raising HDL level. Beside statins, gemfibrozil (loped) and a new drug fenofibrate (Tricor) are also prescribed.

Q.   Should one have statin if he has normal cholesterol?

The statin drugs are used to lower the LDL (bad cholesterol) level. High levels of LDL cholesterol can lead to heart disease. If LDL cholesterol is not high, one need not take statin. A study nicknamed JUPITER was recently conducted on 17,802 people from 26 countries. The men were 50 and over and the women were 60 and over—the ages when cardiovascular risk begins to rise. Participants had no history of heart attacks or strokes, and their LDL cholesterol levels were below 130 mg/dl. It was found that the statin drug rosuvastatin (Crestor) reduced the rate of heart attacks and strokes in people with normal LDL cholesterol who had elevated levels of C-reactive protein (CRP). CRP is a marker of inflammation, and there is increasing evidence that low-grade inflammation raises heart risk.

According to the Framingham Heart Study ongoing since the 1940s the   high levels of HDLs are connected to a lower risk of heart disease. As long as your HDL (good cholesterol) is high enough, you are least at the risk of having a heart disease and need not to take any prescription. It shows that raising HDL can reduce the risk of coronary disease regardless of LDL cholesterol. That is because HDL removes LDL from the arteries and sends it to the liver. And it is the plaque buildup that really causes heart disease and heart attacks – not the cholesterol. Prolonged use of statins causes side effects. Its use for three weeks may cause pain in your legs for which you may take brufen. This may damage your liver and you have to take drugs for it. So, you become drug dependent. It is wise to control your cholesterol without drugs.

Q.   How can level of HDL cholesterol be raised?

A.   To beat the heart disease without drugs, here are five ways to naturally boost your HDL:

1.   Take enough B-3. It is also called as niacin and has been found to raise HDL levels by as much as 24 percent. The best food sources of niacin are liver, chicken, beef, avocados, tomatoes and nuts. You may also take 500 mg of sustained release niacin as a supplement every day. Consult your doc-

tor before taking it.

2.   Take good fat - fish, poultry, nuts, olives, eggs and avocados are all rich in good fats. Cod liver oil – the best omega-3 supplement – will boost your HDL levels naturally.

3.   Give your heart the nutrition it needs with protein. Replace starchy carbohydrates like bread, pasta with high-quality protein which will lower your triglycerides and raise your HDL. The best protein sources are nuts, eggs, poultry, beef and salmon.

4.   Give your hart a workout-- Your heart, just like any muscle in your body needs to be challenged in order to become stronger. The best way to do this is with short-duration, progressive exercises. Walking out side or on the tread mill may increase your heart beat and your heart gets accustomed to take some extra load. Exercise raises your HDL.

5.   Enjoy a drink – Taking two alcohol drinks a day, decrease cholesterol

level, increase antioxidants and reduce level of fibrinogen, a clot-

producing protein.

Q.   What do trans fats do to the heart?
A.   They are chiefly responsible for a condition called atherosclerosis where fatty deposits collect on the inner lining of the arteries and cause the formation of the atheroma* which obstructs free flow of blood in the artery. The plaque contains largely LDL cholesterol. They come from fatty foods. Trans fats are also known to induce inflammation, which initiates plaque formation. According to the World Health Organization not more than one percent of our calories should come from trans fats and less than 10 percent should come from saturated fats. Looking to the harm caused by the trans fats, some governments are planning to ban all trans-fat use in food industry. Food

manufacturers argue that it may be possible to replace trans fats by frying, but people like confectionary products having trans fats. With the ban lots of items including biscuits and pastries will disappear from the market.

Q. **What should we find on the food labels?**
A. You find the amounts of ingredients on the food labels. It may show the amount of cholesterol present in the food, but it is not sufficient. It should be mandatory to describe the amount of trans fats, saturated, monounsaturated and polyunsaturated and total fats. It is also true that if people are very focused on trans fats they may not purchase foods containing them.

Q. **what can I do to reduce my trans fats consumption?**
A. Eat most of the time at home. People, who often eat out, eat less healthy food. Polish people spend only 5 percent of their income on eating out while

* Degeneration of the artery walls.

Americans spend up to 35 percent in restaurants. Michael Pollen the author of "The Omnivore's Dilemma" relates it with obesity. Butter contains trans fats and saturated fats. Replace it with unsaturated fats. Do not eat meat having fat, instead eat lean meat. Pastries, chocolate biscuits and some other confectionary products have high levels of saturated fats, so avoid them. Instead eat more of fruits and vegetables, which have good effect on the body and help reduce the body fat. Eat whole grain bread, porridge, oats and roasted muesli. Some of the low-fat sweet's beverages are fruit ice, fruit pie, and homemade cake, homemade cookies, rasgulla, sandesh, pudding and low-fat yogurt.

Q. **Is low cholesterol level also harmful?**
A. Mostly people focus on high cholesterol level. Low level of cholesterol has not attracted much attention. Recent findings link low cholesterol to certain types of strokes. Men with cholesterol levels below 160 had greater risk of a hemorrhagic stroke (rupturing the blood vessels). Low cholesterol level may also

lead to higher risk of cancer as compared to those with very high cholesterol. Cholesterol is synthesized in our body and is utilized in making cell membranes and hormones. Thus, optimum quantity of it is essential for our body. According to Dr.Michael Oliver, "if too much cholesterol is lost from the cell membrane, it loses the immune resistance" and further reports that older people with low cholesterol level have greater risk of cancer. In a recent study the patients with cholesterol level in the range of 160-220 had fewer deaths from all causes than those having lower or higher cholesterol levels.

Q.   Are diabetes and high cholesterol level related?
A.   Diabetes is considered to be a genetic disposition. People with this predisposition eventually develop diabetes. In most cases before expression of diabetic symptoms, the blood picture often shows high LDL cholesterol and triglyceride levels, low HDL- cholesterol level, high blood pressure and higher risk factor for plaque formation. Once diabetes is established, probability for silent heart attack, peripheral artery disease and stroke is increased.

Q.   Are plant sterols good for heart?
A.   Plant sterols block cholesterol absorption in the gut. 12 to 15 percent decrease in LDL cholesterol has been recorded after taking 2-gram plant sterols for 2-3 weeks. They are known as functional foods and are added to margarines and other such preparations.

Q.   What determines the level of LDL cholesterol in the blood?
A.   LDL cholesterol is synthesized in the liver and is poured in to the blood stream. It is also removed from the blood with the help of LDL cholesterol receptors present on the liver cells surface. When the number of such receptors is decreased the liver, cells are unable to absorb adequate amount of LDL cholesterol, hence there is an increase of it in the blood. Heredity and diet are also responsible to some extent. If it is a hereditary disorder,

then receptors for LDL cholesterol on liver cells are too less or they are completely absent. Such people develop heart ailment at early adulthood. Habit of taking food rich in fats raises LDL cholesterol level.

Q.   Is cow ghee good for heart?
A.   Cow's milk and ghee are considered as most wholesome as they are superior in protein, fat, carbohydrates, vitamins and minerals. Cow's ghee has been used in Indian diet for centuries without any reports of adverse effects on health. Its saturated fat & primarily contains short chain fatty acids, which are not harmful if taken in small quantity. Any adverse finding against cow's ghee is largely due to its consumption in large quantity. Doctors these days allow heart patient's one tea spoonful of cow's ghee in one day.

Q.   How can LDL cholesterol level be decreased in the blood?
A.   Restrict to diet free of saturated fats. Increase in take of unrefined grains. Eat more fruits and vegetables. Increase physical activity and follow the measures described to increase in HDL level.

3.   SMOKING

- Smokers are almost twice as likely to have a heart attack compared with people who have never smoked.
- Smoking increases the risk of developing cardio-vascular diseases which includes coronary heart disease and stroke.
- Smoking damages the lining of your arteries, leading to a build-up of fatty material called atheroma which narrows the artery. This can cause angina, a heart attack or a stroke.
- The carbon monoxide in tobacco smoke reduces the amount of oxygen in your blood. This means your heart has to pump harder to supply the body with the oxygen it

needs.

■   The nicotine in cigarettes stimulates your body to produce adrenaline, which makes your heart beat faster and raises your blood pressure, making your heart work harder.

■   Your blood is more likely to clot, which increases your risk of having a heart attack or stroke. .
    ○   Why Quit?
    ○   Risk to your heart health decreases significantly soon after you stop.

■   By quitting you'll be improving your own health by dramatically reducing your risk of coronary heart disease, stroke and a variety of cancers. You'll feel better, and have more money to spend on other things that you enjoy.
    ○   Second hand smoke
    ○   When non-smokers breathe in second hand smoke - also known as passive smoking - it can be harmful. Research shows that exposure to second hand tobacco smoke is a cause of heart disease in non-smokers, which means you could be harming the health of your children, partner and friends.

4.   Diabetes

The most common cause of heart diseases in a person with diabetes is hardening of the coronary arteries or atherosclerosis, which is a build-up of cholesterol in the blood vessels that supply oxygen and nutrition to the heart.

When the cholesterol plaques can break apart or rupture, the body tries to repair the plaque rupture by sending platelets to seal it up. Because the artery is small, the platelets could block the flow of blood, not allowing for oxygen delivery and a heart attack develops. The same process can happen in all of the arteries in the body, resulting in lack of blood to the brain, causing a stroke or lack of blood to the feet, hands, or arms causing peripheral vascular disease.

Not only are people with diabetes at higher risk for heart disease, they're also at higher risk for heart failure, a serious medical condition in which the heart is unable to pump blood adequately. This can lead to fluid build-up in the lungs that causes difficulty breathing, or fluid retention in other parts of the body (especially the legs) that causes swelling.

DIET

Longevity and quality of our life depend entirely on what we eat. Healthy person feels fit, energetic and has better mind set and can enjoy a life better. Inactive life with improper feeding habits leads to diseases like obesity which is responsible for hypertension and heart problems. Many diets have been suggested for losing weight having underlined idea to have good quality of food in appropriate amount along with suitable exercise. Our food consists mainly of carbohydrates, proteins, fats, vitamins and minerals. The following account describes the physiological importance of the various food ingredients.

CARBOHYDRATES

Carbohydrates or Carbs we get mainly from cereals, vegetables and fruits in the form of sugar and starch. They contain carbon, hydrogen and oxygen. Our digestive system breaks them down into sugars which are absorbed by the blood, and a part of which are stored in the liver as glycogen - the reserved energy and the rest is utilized in body functions. Carbohydrates may be classified as simple and complex carbohydrates.

Simple carbohydrates—their chemical structure is simple, so they are easily digested and converted into glucose or blood sugar. Natural simple carbohydrates we get from potatoes, sweet potatoes, whole grain bread and cereals. We also eat simple carbohydrates as wheat flour and refined sugar. During the process of refining, fiber, fat and micronutrients get removed from the original product. They are therefore not considered as good carbs.

Complex carbohydrates—their chemical structure is complex so they take more time to break into sugars in the digestive system. Such sugars form a long-term energy pool in our body. Plant food that we eat consists of complex crabs, fiber, plant-based fats and other nutrients. They are also known as good carb or healthiest natural food because of the nutritious ingredients and slow break down. The fiber cannot be broken down by our digestive enzymes so they pass out of the body system without being absorbed. Fiber makes the bulk of the faecal matter and helps in passing out of the bowel. There are some soluble fibers also (as in oats) which are assimilated in our system and help control LDL cholesterol.

During the last century there has been tremendous progress in producing variety of food products with new combinations to make them more appealing and tastier. Many diets are being recommended for slimming/ losing weight by restricting carbohydrates but most of them pose threat to health. Preparing white bread with refined wheat flour depletes it of the bran which provides the fiber, and wheat germ which is rich in vitamin B. Such foods having high glycemic index increases the sugar level. The pancreas has to secrete more insulin to deal with the extra load of sugar and this extra insulin may enhance the triglycerides and cholesterol level. A study from 1984 to 1996 on 74000 women showed that high consumption of refined diet increased triglyceride levels and reduced good cholesterol (HDL)resulting in high blood pressure and inflammation and possibility of plaque formation in the arteries. High carbohydrate diet causes craving for food which induces nibbling all the time. Eating fats and protein along with carbohydrates limits the sugar level, so there is no craving for food. Hydrogenation of vegetable oils causes depletion of essential fatty acids which are good for our system. Sweets with saccharin and cyclamate, macaroni, white flour products, all lack essential nutrients, moreover, they contain preservatives and other harmful substances like pesticides and detergents which have adverse effects on our system. In fact, fungi and bacteria like the same substances which we like; therefore, the manufacturers remove or modify the substances liked by fungi and bacteria to increase the shelf-life of their products.

If you deplete vegetables, whole grain and fruits from your diet your heart does not get every day protectors like soluble fiber, minerals, vitamins and antioxidants. If your diet has low carbohydrate and more saturated fats, your heart is at risk. It is therefore recommended that for losing weight a diet with moderate carbohydrates along with fruits, vegetables and whole grain is much better than a low carb diet.

FATS:

Fats are formed of carbon, hydrogen and oxygen. They may be solid or liquid. They are important ingredient of our food which we get from animal and plant sources and play a vital role in our body.

1. They are concentrated stored source of energy.
2. They provide insulation under our skin to protect the body from extreme
heat and cold.
3. They provide protection to our internal organs.

A fat molecule consists of one molecule of glycerol and three molecules
of fatty acids, therefore, also called triglycerides. Fats break down to form fatty acids which are essential for body functions. They are important structural components of the cell membrane and serve as substrate for the synthesis of a variety of secretions including potent hormones. When energy is required, these fatty acids break down forming carbon dioxide, water, heat and energy.

Fats are of two types:

Saturated fats -All fatty acids consist of a chain of carbon atoms with varying number of hydrogen atoms attached to them. A molecule that has two hydrogen atoms attached to each carbon atom is said to be saturated, because it is holding all the hydrogen atoms it possibly can.

Unsaturated fatty acids-- A fatty acid which has a missing pair of hydrogen atoms on one of its carbon atoms is called monounsaturated fatty acid. If more than two hydrogen atoms are missing, it is called polyunsaturated fatty acid. A lot of medical attention has been paid to saturated and unsaturated fatty acids as they are held responsible for atherosclerosis and heart failure.

Essential fatty acids: Three fatty acids namely linolic acid, linolenic acid and arachidonic acid are known as essential fatty acids as they facilitate the breakdown of saturated fats and cholesterol, thus preventing them from depositing in the arteries. They are obtained from vegetable oils like ground nut oil, olive oil, soya oil etc.

PROTEINS

These are building molecules of the body, required to compensate the loss due to daily wear and tear of the tissues, for the formation of new tissues in children, wound healing, synthesis of enzymes, some hormones and plasma membrane. These are complex molecules formed by combination of amino acids. Proteins that we take in our meals are broken down into amino acids which recombine to form the required proteins. Twenty different amino acids accomplish this task. Ten of them are essential amino acids which are not synthesized in our body and the other ten are synthesized in the body with the help of carbohydrate and fat derivatives.

Proteins which contain all the ten essential amino acids (animal proteins like egg, milk, meat and fish) are considered as first-class proteins. Gelatin although an animal protein is considered as second-class protein as is vegetable proteins, since they do not contain all the ten essential amino acids. Amino acid composition of our body proteins closely resembles the amino acid composition of our food. This facilitates synthesis of body proteins without much energy expenditure. Such proteins are known as proteins of high biological value. Mother's milk has higher biological value than cow's milk, although both have high biological value. Lesser amount of such food is required. Mostly we eat food of mixed biological value. Protein requirement of an average person is 0.8gm/kg body weight. As such a man weighing 70kg requires only 56gm of protein. Excess food protein consumption has no advantage to the body, because excess amino acids formed may lead to positive nitrogen balance resulting in proteinaceous deposits in tissues.   Indian population is largely vegetarian. Non-vegetarians also eat vegetarian food most of the time. In western countries protein in the food comes mainly from animal sources like meat, fish and eggs, but in India people get most of it from milk and milk products including butter, *desi* ghee, curd, "*khoya*", and "*paneer*". Milk is considered to be better source of protein as compared to the plant proteins. Traditionally, children in India are grown on milk (and milk products) which is considered as complete food as it provides protein, carbohydrates, fat, vitamins A and D, calcium, magnesium, phosphorus and potassium. Poor people find it difficult to afford milk for their children, leading to protein deficiency and malnutrition as well as vitamin A deficiency (a cause of blindness).

Since milk has up to 8% fat, heart patients should not consume whole milk, instead low-fat milk should be used for drinking and curd preparation. Food items containing high fat, cheese, cream, ghee, ice cream should be avoided; instead butter milk should be preferred.

FIBER

With the changing pattern of life, we are forgetting valuable aspects of our food for the sake of convenience. Traditionally our food consisted of recipes of whole grain, milk and curd which have now been replaced by bread, butter and coffee. Younger generation prefers fast food made from refined material. Our fiber intake has considerably reduced. Fibers are important components of all parts of plants. We ingest them in grains, fruits and vegetables. Most of the fibers are not digested yet they help in maintaining our health. In the digestive tract they absorb water, become soft and swell. They bind the undigested food material and help in easy transport of waste material through bowel. They absorb excess fat and cholesterol, thus protecting arteries from plaque formation. Also, they increase the tone of the colon, help in bowel movement, and keep away constipation, piles and stomach cancer. Foods like egg, meat, fish and milk products do not have fiber. Two types of fiber are found:

1.   Water insoluble fiber - They include cellulose, lignin and many hemicelluloses. Found in cereals, unprocessed fruits, they help in cleaning bowel as described above. They help in weight loss, as they give a sense of filling for a longer period and holding water in the gut.

2.   Water soluble fiber- Found in apple, banana and many other fruits, barley, oat and nuts, they include gums, pectin, mucilage, some hemicelluloses and polysaccharides. Oats are rich source of manganese, selenium, tryptophan along with soluble fiber (beta glucan). We need 25-30 grams of fiber every day, but we get only 20grams from normal diet. It is therefore, recommended that 10% fiber supple-

ment should come from fruits, vegetables and nuts. Those with heart problem may increase the fiber consumption gradually (but in limits) with the advice of the doctor and should not take fiber as alternate to drugs. By way of keeping your alimentary canal clean, fiber helps in maintaining good mood.

Too much of fiber is harmful

•	Excessive fiber in the diet is also harmful, as it may produce gas and cause bloating. Moderate intake of fluid is necessary for proper utilization of fiber in the gut. One should adjust fiber as per his/her body response. This can be done by increasing fiber intake till no adverse effects are seen.

•	They may bind with the minerals and reduce absorption by the gut.

•	Oat is a good source of fiber but at the same time its fat content is rather more. It may, therefore, increase fat consumption; however, oat bran has low fat content.

FREQUENTLY ASKED QUESTIONS

Q. How dietary fiber help in lowering cholesterol level?

A. A part of cholesterol synthesized in the liver is used for the synthesis of bile, which helps in digestion of the food. After digestion of food, bile is reabsorbed by the liver for further use, which may increase the level of cholesterol. Dietary fiber disrupts this cycle and absorbs the bile from the alimentary canal and passes it out of the body with the faecal matter. In this way amount of cholesterol available in the liver is reduced which otherwise would form bad cholesterol harmful for the heart. Soluble fibers reduce total cholesterol by 7.0% and LDL by 5%, thereby reducing the heart risk by 10-15 percent.

Q. How they help in control of diabetes?

A. Since they have low glycemic index (slow glucose absorption), they increase glucose tolerance and maintain blood glucose level.

Q. How dietary fiber intake may be increased?

A. White bread, pizza, patties, noodles etc have low fiber content. In place of white bread brown bread should be preferred. It's better to bank upon wheat porridge, oats with curds and fruits and sprouts in breakfast. Meals should include whole wheat flour *chapattis* with *dal*, vegetables and salad.

Q. What are the important sources of fiber?

A. Important sources of fiber may be seen in the table.

Table: Showing different grades of fiber content in food items.

Low	Noodles, all-purpose flour, rice, potato, sago, fruit juice
Medium	Wheat, maize, bajra, chick peas, pears, beet root, turnip, radish, some varieties of rice
High	Oat, barley, white millet, ragi, soybean, black gram, kidney beans, beans, peas, apple, guava, grapes, peach, apricot.

Sprouts—they contain largest amount of nutrients per unit. They provide good amount of enzymes and vitamins. In early sprouting time the vitamin C value of wheat increases 600 times. The wheat germ juice is good for fighting the body ailments. Vitamin B in sprouted seeds increases by 1000 folds. For sprouting wheat, green gram (moong dal), peas, barley, bajra, gram, beans, ground nut, fenugreek and Alfaalfa seeds are usually recommended. One cup (about 33 g) of sprout gives 1mg dietary fiber, 2mg sodium, 1g carbohydrate, 1gprotein and 08 calories.

Q.   What is muesli and how is it beneficial?

**A.   **Muesli is a porridge made from oats, cereals, fruits and nuts. It was developed by a Swiss physician more than a hundred years ago for hospital patients. It is now taken in breakfast or in the evening. All the components of it are good for health and help in losing weight. Since it has enough fiber with low glycemic index, it is digested slowly so one doesn't feel like eating for a long time. It may contain sugar also, so while purchasing check the sugar content on the label.

Q   Why eating slowly is advised?

A.   If you eat fast, by the time your body signals that it is full, you have already over eaten. Eating slowly allows you time to chew the food and mix with the saliva which helps in digestion. Eating slow is beneficial for weight loss. Thai food is quite spicy which increases metabolism. Hot spices make you eat slowly. French people enjoy eating leisurely together in the evening. Healthy conversation with slow eating makes you feel full soon.

Q.   Is it true that low carb diet brings about weight fall quickly?

A.   It is true, because when intake of carb is low you largely depend on stored energy i.e., glycogen which when breaks down releases water, so you lose water weight. When you eat fewer calories, you lose weight but this may lead in some to headache or nausea. When you have little carbohydrate available in the body, your fat deposits start depleting. When fats burn without carbs more ketones* and water are formed which cause poor appetite. If ketone level rises in the body, minerals from the bones are depleted causing fragile bones.

Studies show that there is an initial weight loss in group with low carb diet but, over period of few months it has no significant benefit over moderate carb group. It is also found in experiments with different diets that different diets suit different people. Low carb with high fat and protein may raise LDL cholesterol and deprive us of the essential nutrients that we get from vegetables, grains and fruits. In addition, high protein diet may induce diabetes and its consequences. Another study shows that good carbohydrates help in controlling weight. Low carb foods available in the market for taste are loaded with more calories in the form of fats as in pasta, ice cream, pizzas and snack bars. Refined carbohydrates are digested quickly so the sugar level in the blood spikes. More insulin is secreted from the pancreas to absorb extra sugar. This extra insulin induces bad effects on our body organs. It is advised to eat sufficient carbohydrates, protein and fat which keep the blood sugar level steady. Good fats do not increase your LDL cholesterol but maintain HDL level. Poor quality of fats, like saturated fats may deplete HDL cholesterol.

Q.   Is chocolate good for the heart?

A.   Recent study claims that moderate levels of chocolate may be associated with a 33 percent decrease in the risk of developing heart disease. A study published in British Medical Journal shows positive link between eating chocolate and healthy health, giving a nice reprieve to chocoholics.

*Three water soluble molecules produced by liver

Individuals with the highest level of chocolate consumption had a 37 percent decrease in cardiovascular diseases and a 29 percent reduction in stroke. Other studies suggest that dark chocolate is more beneficial because of its higher cocoa content which has useful flavones*.

Q.   How good are almonds for heart health?

A.   Almonds are full of nutrition and are good for the heart and general health. They contain 65-70 % mono and polyunsaturated fats. They reduce C-reactive protein which effects flow of blood in the arteries. They are rich source of potassium, manganese, magnesium and copper and have low sodium. Magnesium has positive effect on blood vessels facilitating smooth flow of nutritious materials to the tissues. Riboflavin and other constituents act as energy booster.

Risk of heart disease is reduced to 50 percent if you take ten almonds for five days a week.

Q.   Is fruit juice good for heart?

A.   Fruit juice contains good sugar, vitamins, minerals and antioxidants which are good for heart and blood vessels, but it has very little dietary fiber. It is better to consume unpeeled fruits (wherever possible). It is not wise to drink large glass of juice; rather it should be taken in small quantity two to three times. Juice may be taken with breakfast, in the noon and afternoon. Grape juice has revere sterol which is good for the blood vessels. Fresh fruit juice is much better than canned juice.

Salt intake:

Sodium is an electrolyte and plays a key role in maintaining water balance in our body. Sodium works to push water into cells while potassium does its job of pushing waste out of cells. This balance helps to prevent dehydration and promotes healthy cell function.

* Are yellow pigments which occur in plant kingdom

In addition to its role in cell health, sodium is required for nerve and muscle function. It is generally believed that high sodium intake may cause high blood pressure. In fact, high sodium in diet holds water in the body fluids. When more sodium is present in the blood, it collects more water which increases blood pressure and the vessel walls come under stress. Our forefathers knew this fact and recommended low salt diet to treat high blood pressure without medicines. In a healthy person sodium is present in the body fluid and potassium in the cells. Excessive sodium forces loss of potassium through urine, creating a condition of potassium deficiency. Both of them working in a balanced way facilitate the inflow and outflow of materials from the cells. When potassium is depleted, more sodium enters the cells and draws more water so the cells become swollen and turgid. Sometimes doctors advise small quantity of potassium to the patients of high blood pressure in place of sodium. In fact, the food items that we eat already have enough sodium, to the tune that one can do without taking extra sodium.

Table: Sodium and potassium contents of some food items (Mg/100 g edible portion)

Food Item	Sodium	Potassium

Processed cheese	290-400	70
Egg	140	140
Butter	850	28
Hydrogenated oils	4	0
Mutton	33	270
Chicken	100	300
Rohu fish	101	288
Prawns	66	272
Pomfret fish	75	385
Lobster	21	180
Bean sprout	30	840
(mung)	25	1150
Green beans	40	800
Urd dal	28	1104
Tur dal	58	138
Cauliflower	10	110
Cabbage	10	50
Cucumber	3	200
Brinjal	60	256
Coriander leaves	58	206
Spinach	4	127
Onion	13	145
Tomatoes	33	138
Radish	36	88
Banana	--	320
Cherries red	28	75
Apple	10	773
Coconut (tender)	3	80
Grapes	5	91
Guava	--	270
Lemon sour	4.5	93
Orange	1	247
Plum's red	1	133
Pomegranate	6	69
Papaya	8	70

Rice	20	315
Wheat flour(atta)	9.3	130
Wheat flour(	600	178
Maida) Bread	400	158
brown	5	856
Bread white	2	740
Almond	20	770
Ground	10	560
nut(roasted)	2	568
Coconut dry		
Cashew nut		
Walnut		

The minimum requirement of sodium for normal body function is about 500 mg/day, but people consume much more sodium through processed foods and table salt, the recommendation for sodium intake is less than 2,300 mg/day for adults including the salt used in cooking. People diagnosed with high blood pressure or at risk for high blood pressure should limit sodium consumption to 1,500 mg/day.

Some people are in the habit of adding some salt to their food without tasting it. They should taste it first to determine if it is really needed to add more from the shaker. Low level of sodium may also be dangerous. Physically active persons might be in danger of low sodium levels, as prolonged physical activity causes sodium loss through sweating. Initial symptoms of sodium deficiency (also called hyponatremia) are fatigue and confusion, but it can lead to more serious conditions of seizure and even coma and death. Those taking mostly fresh foods and large amounts of water may take in little sodium.

Many of the processed foods have good amount of sodium, excess calories, saturated and trans-fats and preservatives. It is best to limit the consumption of these foods to maintain proper amount of sodium. There are of course some processed foods that fit into healthy diet and also provide some sodium. Develop the habit of reading food labels to ensure that you stay under the daily limit of 2,300 mg. Salted nuts provide healthy fats, protein and fiber along with sodium.

Q.   Is it true that oats are good for heart?

A.   Oats are high in soluble fiber which binds with the bad LDL cholesterol (LDL). Eating oats regularly can lower blood cholesterol by 20 percent. Also oats have low glycemic index and help you lose weight since they release energy slowly, stabilizing blood sugar and inducing burning of fats.

Q.   Is coffee good for heart?

A   Coffee was once suspected to cause many diseases. It is now believed to help in lowering the risk of type-2 diabetes, Gall stones, Parkinson's disease, Cirrhosis and certain types of cancers. It has many antioxidants which protect the heart and reduce the risk of cardiovascular disease. Black coffee is even better. A Norwegian study showed that a cup of brewed coffee is much better than fruit juice. Dieticians suggest that up to two cups of coffee a day without sugar and whole milk is good. Excessive drinking of coffee may induce dehydration or may raise blood pressure. Unfiltered coffee contains more cholesterol raising substance-cafestol, so those having high cholesterol level should prefer instant coffee.

Q.   Can a patient with cardiovascular disease take desighee?

A.   *Desi* ghee has high calorie content and is rich in saturated fat. One tea spoon ghee made of cow's milk may be taken, but not as cooking medium. Recently it has been described different from other saturated fats.

Q.   Which oil should be used for cooking?

A.   No single oil can be said to be perfect as their nutritive content vary. It is recommended that either blends of two – three oils be used or different oil be used every time. Blends may be (1) canola oil with rice bran and sunflower oil, (2) sunflower oil with ground nut oil, and (3) different grades of olive oil. For minimizing the oil consumption, nonstick utensils should be used.

Q.   Can bakery products be consumed?

A.   Bakery products are prepared generally with hydrogenated vegetable oils having saturated fats along with trans-fats, which increase cholesterol level. Better to avoid them. Instead, homemade snacks should be preferred, that too after blotting off the oil.

Q.   Can spicy food be taken?

A.   All spices have some beneficial effects, but they should be used in the amount just to make the food palatable. Spicy foods generally have more fat which should be avoided.

Q.   Indian cuisine also includes chutneys, pickles and papads. Are they allowed to a heart patient?

A.   Commercial pickles and papads contain more salt, spices and preservatives. It is better to have homemade pickles and chutneys like that of green coriander, mint and garlic specially made for heart patient. Onion in vinegar is good. Roasted papads should be preferred over fried ones.

Q.   What type of sweets can be taken?

A.   Sweets made from skimmed milk with low sugar may be taken. Rasgullas, sandesh and other such preparations may be taken. Khoya preparations and fried sweets should be completely avoided.

Q.   How much tea, coffee and beverages may be taken?

A.   For a normal person up to 5 cups of tea and 2 cups of coffee are alright. Cardiac patients should avoid excessive use of coffee containing products. Two cups of tea and two cups of coffee may be taken. Colas generally contain caffeine; they should be taken in limit; Instead, juice of citrus fruits or curd preparations should be preferred.

Q.   What type of food may be taken in parties?

A.   Parties generally offer food rich in fat and spices. It is better to take a smaller plate and instead of curries, pieces should be taken, that too in small servings which should not be repeated. Oily preparations should be avoided. Salad, curd and plain rice may be taken. Sweets may be taken in very small quantity.

Q.   Which vegetables are good for heart patients?

A.   Green leafy vegetables are healthy but they should be properly washed before cooking. Some vegetables interfere with the drugs. People taking acetron should avoid leafy vegetables containing more potassium, especially of cabbage family.

Q.   How good are dry fruits for heart patients?

A.   Dry fruits are rich in monounsaturated fats and vitamin E. They are also calorie rich. Those who need to reduce calorie intake should avoid dry fruits.

Q.   Is fish oil a substitute of fish?

A.   Fish oil is not a substitute of fish. Taking fish oil in small quantity is good, but high intake may affect the blood clotting mechanism which may lead to internal bleeding in case of accident. Eskimos consume more fish oil and are known for nose bleeding, which may be fatal. Fish muscle has more nutrients. Addition of fish to regular diet reduces the consumption of other meats and poultry products which are rich in saturated fatty acids. Fish is a fairly satiety food but fish oil is not, it rather increases one's calorie intake. Taking fish three times a week is good for heart patients.

Q.   How is omega 3s beneficial?

A.   Omega 3s is known to reduce inflammation and blood clot in the coronary arteries. They keep the nerve cells healthy, as a result of which heart and blood vessels remain properly toned up.

Q.   Are eggs responsible for heart attack?

A.   Eggs are very nutritious. They are the prime source of vitamin D and also provide vitamin A, B_2, B_{12} and E. Eating three eggs a week is quite safe. Excessive consumption of eggs should be avoided.

Q.   Can diet actually help to clear the existing plaque?

A.   There is sufficient scientific evidence that supports the notion that post heart attack patients should adapt to recommended style of diet, be physically active through exercise and should not smoke. The Lyon Heart Study which tested Mediterranean diet in cardiac patients found it to be able to reduce the recurrence of heart attack by 70% compared to the normal diet. Yoga exercises along with proper diet are claimed to clear existing plaques.

Q.   In festival days how one should hold himself from unwanted food?

A.   Festivals come with mouthwatering dishes. Overindulgence may cause health problems; hence one has to balance his desire for feasting with a healthy choice. Food researchers and health experts have found that right choice of cooking oil and strict eating discipline can help you in enjoying festivals. Festival cuisines in India are predominantly oil based which is associated with high calorie content. The key to healthy cooking is to select less absorbing cooking oil. It should be ascertained that it does not stick to the utensil. The low absorption oil makes the food lighter which is easier to digest and it contains essential nutrients like vitamin A and D.

Besides what you eat, it is important to consider how you eat and how much you eat. It is better to consume smaller proportions of sweets and fried preparations. Some tips are:

•	Do not surrender to offerings. Gently say "I shall help myself".

•	Take larger proportions of fruits and salad.

•	Drink a glass of water before you eat.

•	While preparing cookies at home ensure that your preparations are not too heavy and easy to digest. opt for low fat milk and avoid sugar, better to use natural sweeteners like dates and honey.

•	Do not overcook your food.

•	You can brush your stuff with oil and bake in oven.

Table: showing preferred and worth avoiding food items.

Prefer	Avoid
Butter milk, fresh fruit juice, lemon water or	Canned fruit juice

lemon soda	
Fresh or frozen fruit	Fruits with cream or ice cream
Fresh frozen vegetables cooked with minimum quantity of unsaturated fat	Vegetables cooked in vanaspati ghee, butter or with added cream
High fat cheese	Low fat cheese
Rasogulla, Sandesh et.	Khoya sweets, pudding with ice cream
Corn without oil	Fried snacks
Yogurt	High fat curd
Skimmed / low fat milk	Whole milk
Idli	Dosa, pizza etc.

Table: showing important nutrients in food items

Food Items	You Get
Dark leafy vege-tables	Vitamin A and C, foliate, beta carotene and fiber
Beans	Fiber, protein and iron
Sweet potato	Vitamin A, C and fiber
Dark berries	Vitamin C iron and fiber
Whole grains	Fiber, vitamin B and E, Zink and Selenium
Nuts	Protective oils, fiber and vitamins
Yogurt Salmon, tuna and other cold-water fishes	Protein, Calcium, Phosphorus and omega-3 fatty acids

EXERCISE AND THE HEART

Regular exercise can improve the cardiovascular fitness at any age. Some types of exercises are more effective than others. Aerobics or any other exercise that work body's large muscles for at least 20 minutes, increase cardiac output and metabolic rate. Three to five sessions a week are recommended for heart health. Brisk walking, running, bicycling, swimming are examples of aerobic activities. Regular exercise increases oxygen demand of the muscles. For this adequate cardiac output and respiratory efficiency is necessary which can be achieved by exercising for 2-3 weeks. This allows maximum oxygen delivery to the tissues. Oxygen delivery also rises, because with exercise the muscles develop more capillary network. If you have undergone balloon angioplasty, bypass surgery or have angina, you must take regular physical activity under the instructions of your doctor. By exercising a heart patient also boosts his confidence, increases fitness level, cuts risk of dying and overcomes depression, stress and social isolation. Regular exercise also reduces blood pressure and anxiety. It also controls body weight and increases the body's ability to dissolve the blood clots by increasing thrombolytic activity.

An athlete undergoes strenuous training and can achieve cardiac output double that of a non-exercising person, because of the heart enlargement. Even in such cases despite a larger heart the cardiac output at rest is the same as that of a normal untrained person, because stroke volume is increased while heart rate is decreased. The resting heart rate of a trained athlete is often 40 to 60 beats per minute (resting bradycardia).

Some of the exercises are outlined here under:

AEROBICS

Aerobic exercise is crucial for heart patients. To prevent monotony, take a mix of exercises; for instance, walking briskly one day and going for a bike ride the next. When the weather is bad, indoors work out may be taken like stair-climbing or treadmill walking.

Start your aerobic program slowly and try to build up to at least 30 minutes three times a week. The 30 minutes need not to be all at once, one can break them into two or three sessions, depending on your physical condition. Before you begin aerobic exercises, warm up by stretching or walking around for about five minutes; after your session, cool down the same way. Ask your doctor to recommend a safe exercise, safe heart rate, and check your rate as you workout. Electronic pedometer is now available which records the time, your total steps, speed and calories you burn

For older people brisk walk for 30 minutes is a must. In due course it proves to be holding your strength for a longer period. A study was made on 220 old people near about retirement age. Half of them had brisk walk for 30 minutes and the other half did not exercise. After one year there was 12 percent increase in aerobic power of exercise group along with more strength and hip flexibility as compared to non-exercising group. Aerobic exercises improve the power of lungs and the heart, which helps in maintaining muscle strength and bone density.

STRENGTH TRAINING

With the help of a physiotherapist develop a regimen suitable for your needs, taking into account your age, weight and physical condition.

Strength training helps you build up various parts of your body by using resistance. It improves metabolism, and you burn calories for some time even if you do not exercise. You may use weight machines, hand weights, resistance bands or simply your own weight. Heart patients usually start with low resistance and work up to a higher level. An example of a strength exercise is an arm raise. Sit in an armless chair with your feet flat on the ground about hip-distance apart and your hands hanging at your sides. Hold a weight in each hand with your palms facing in. Lift your arms straight to the sides until they are parallel to the ground. Hold for a few second, and then slowly relax your arms. Do it ten times. After few days weight on the arms may be increased.

A study made in America suggests that muscle and bone loss could be stopped and even reversed through weight training. Postmenopausal women under 60 when lifted weights twice a week for one year, showed an increase in bone density and strength test also showed beneficial effects. Combination of aerobics and weight training exercise can control blood sugar to some extent.

FLEXIBILITY

Flexibility exercises are the third important component for cardiac patients. Stretching strengthens, relaxes your muscles and improves your range of motion. The American Heart Association recommends stretching all parts of your body.

A simple one is neck stretch. Sit straight on a chair with your feet hip-distance apart. Without moving your back or shoulders, slowly rotate your head around to look over your right shoulder. Return to center and repeat on the left. Do it ten times.

ALCOHOL AND HEART

There is a very clear link between regularly drinking too much alcohol and having high blood pressure. Over time, high blood pressure (hypertension) puts strain on the heart muscle and can lead to cardiovascular disease which increases your risk of heart attack and stroke.

Those who drink regularly and consume more than the lower risk guidelines are likely to be advised to cut down or stop drinking completely.

If you already have a condition that causes arrhythmias, alcohol may increase that risk. This can be especially dangerous in those who have inherited heart rhythm conditions.

Heavier drinking (binge drinking) can also bring on a first episode of arrhythmia; once this has happened for the first time, you're at an increased risk in the future.

When you stop drinking, or reduce the amount you drink, you'll see rapid improvement in your blood pressure (you should see a reduction within a few days).

If you have alcoholic cardiomyopathy, stopping drinking can lead to improvement or even recovery for many.

IS ALCOHOL GOOD FOR MY HEART?

There is no drink, such as red wine or beer that can be proven 'better' than another.

It is safest not to drink regularly more than 14 units per week, to keep health risks from drinking alcohol to a low level, and that if you do drink as much as 14 units per week, it is best to spread this evenly over 3 days or more.

Drinking alcohol to excess can cause other serious health conditions, such as cardiomyopathy (where the heart muscle is damaged and can't work as efficiently as it used to) and arrhythmias (abnormal heart rhythms). Some of these conditions can increase your risk of stroke.

Overall, the risks far outweigh any possible benefits.

There is certainly no reason to start drinking alcohol if you don't already. There is also no drink, such as red wine or beer that can be proven 'better' than another.

SLEEP AND HEART PROBLEM

Sleep is an important component of healthy life. Insufficient sleep keeps us feeling dull, the next day. We feel weak, our face does not glow and dark circles may appear under our eyes. It leads to bad mood, lowered body resistance and weight gain. Adequate sleep is crucial for proper brain function as air is necessary for respiration. Not getting sufficient sleep may also cause serious consequences like diabetes, hypertension, heart problem, obesity and memory loss. Brain needs time to sift and erase the events of the day and clean its hard drive to create space for the next day's events. Researchers have found that too little sleep may induce more calcium build up in arteries of the heart. A study made on 495 participants aged 35 to 47 years, 27% of those getting less than five hours of sleep showed plaques in their heart blood vessels, while 11% subjects sleeping for recommended five to seven hours also had plaques. Only 6% subjects sleeping for more than seven hours did not show such development.

Earlier studies were inconclusive because the investigators relied upon the accounts about sleep as given by the subjects. In a recent study at Chicago University the subjects wore a wrist monitor which recorded activity at 30 seconds interval. When the monitor was quite the subject was asleep. This gave exact timing of sleeping. When we talk to a cardiologist, we mention other symptoms but not the sleep. It is now suggested that doctors and patients should consider sleep also in addition to other parameters such as high cholesterol, hypertension and diabetes.

It is claimed that an additional sleep of one hour was equivalent to lowering of systolic blood pressure by 16.5mm/Hg. Experts are not very clear about how the sleep is an issue in formation of the plaque. One explanation suggests inflammation may be responsible. Too little sleep may raise the cortisol level which induces inflammation that may help in formation of the plaque, which can block the blood vessels of heart or brain leading to heart attack or stroke. Also, too little sleep may increase the level of fight or flight hormone (adrenalin) which is responsible for stress and higher heart rate. If it continues chronically, it may harm the heart.

Sleeplessness makes you forgetful: brain events called "sharp waves" are responsible for consolidating memory. These ripples also transfer learned information from the hippocampus* to the cortex of the brain for future use as long-term memory. Sharp wave ripples occur mostly during deepest level of sleep.

Q. What should be the optimum period of sleep?

A. It is recommended that one should take six to eight hours sleep.

Q. Is sleeping too much harmful?

A. The studies show that people who sleep more than eight hours a night may be more likely to have chest pain or angina or coronary artery disease due to narrowing of blood vessels that supply blood and oxygen to the heart. A study made by Prof. Lion Lack of Flinder's University, Australia suggests that if you sleep two hours longer on weekends, your body clock gets delayed by 45 minutes. So, you are less sleepy on Sunday night, which will keep you tired the next day. To compensate this two-hour sleep, better you have a nap on Sunday afternoon. If, however you oversleep, get up and be for a while in the early Sun.

Q. What makes people to sleep longer?

A. Sleeping too much may be associated to socio economic circumstances. A recent study on more than 140000 participants showed that sleep disturbance on at least three nights a week is associated with obesity, diabetes myocardial infarction, coronary artery disease and stroke. Smoking cigarettes harm the heart in a way that it damages the blood vessel's function, thereby decreasing their elasticity and increasing the risk of hardening of the vessels (Atherosclerosis). Sleep is also associated with weight gain. Lack of sleep is related to increase in hunger and appetite and possibly to obesity. According to a 2004 study people who sleep less than six hrs. a day were 30% more likely to become obese than those who slept for seven hrs. or more. There is a link between sleep and certain peptides. Ghrelin stimulates hunger and leptin sends signals to brain to suppress appetite. Short sleep time decreases leptin and increases ghrelin. Sleep loss also develops craving for high fat and high carbohydrate foods. Lack of sleep can affect interpretation of events as a result of which there is decrease in ability to make sound judgment, we are unable to

* Small organ located within the brain & is chiefly associated with long term memory.

assess situations accurately and act wisely. Sleep loss for days together may cause appearance of fine lines and dark circles under the eyes. Lesser sleep causes release of cortisol (stress hormone) in excess amount which can breakdown skin collagen- the protein that keeps the skin smooth and elastic. Sleep loss and depression feed each other. Sleep loss causes depression and depression can make it more difficult to fall asleep. Treating sleep problem can help in ameliorating depression.

Q. How to correct the sleep disorder?

A. Relieving stress is the best way to get healthy sleep. Our body and brain need time to relax. Go for jogging, bicycling and swimming for half an hour. Tired you shall get better and deep sleep. Make your bed room more comfortable. It should be quite and airy. If using an air conditioner, set it at a comfortable temperature. Darken the bed room as far as possible. Use a net or a repellant to ward off the mosquitoes. Taking bath with warm water with lavender oil added can make you sleepy. Take a banana and hot milk with honey before going to sleep. That gives you L-tryptophan which stimulates the brain for sleep. If you wake up early in the morning, do not lay turning in the bed, instead get up and engage yourself in work. After some time when you feel tired, go to sleep again. Try to work on a plan rigidly for getting up and going to bed at fixed timing.

As it is not possible to control every factor that contributes to stress some of the following points may be followed to make the day more productive:

- Schedule the work and find ways to eliminate problems.
- Try to deal with worries much before going to bed.
- Meditate before going to bed.
- Take daily exercise but not within 4 hrs. of bed time. Studies have shown that exercise during the day can improve sleep at night. Exercise increases body temperature, which drops significantly in few hours. This drop in temperature makes it easier for us to fall asleep. Aerobic exercises are very helpful in combating insomnia as they may increase the amount of oxygen in the blood. Ask your doctor as to which exercise will suit your body. Do not go to sleep with full belly because after meals most of the blood flows towards the digestive system. You will feel uncomfortable. Do not take spicy food. It can lead to heart burn. There must be a gap of at least four hours between heavy meal and sleep

time. Proteins are harder to digest, so avoid taking more protein before bed time.

•   Avoid alcohol within 4 hrs. of bedtime. It may help you in falling asleep, but you may experience frequent wakeups. This may cause restless sleep and headache in the morning.

•   It is better to be hydrated throughout the day, but well before bedtime take minimum fluids. Avoid coffee or tea at bedtime. This may interrupt your sleep for urination.

•   Avoid watching TV at bedtime

•   Avoid smoking before bedtime.

•   Listen soft music before going to bed

Sleeping drugs.

There may be many reasons for sleeplessness including psychological or emotional issues, or mild depression. It may also be related to ageing. Sometimes you do not find any reason for sleeplessness. It may be for a short period or may prolong over weeks. People may feel drowsiness during day but are unable to nap, which may cause them to become forgetful and are not able to concentrate on the job. If underlying cause is properly treated, insomnia usually improves. If not improved, people go for sleeping pills. It is found that people aged 60 or more are usually taking pills. Some take it sparingly while others take regularly. Some of the drugs known as sleeping drugs are as follows: -

1.   Ambien (Zolpidem): It is good for getting to sleep, but some people show the tendency to wake up in the middle of the night. Its extended-release version Ambient

CR helps to get sleep in short time. These drugs should be taken when you have seven to eight hours to sleep. An oral spray known as Zolpimist containing active ingredients of Ambien has been approved by the Food and Drug Administration of USA for short term treatment to those who have difficulty in falling asleep. Women are given lower doses as drugs from their body are washed out more slowly than men. The agency recommended that care should be taken in performing activities in the morning which require alertness as the level of drug may be still high in the morning.

2.		Lunesta (Eszopiclone): It also helps in falling asleep quickly and may give seven-to-eight-hour sleep. Full sleep should be taken to avoid grogginess.

3.		Rozerem (Ramelteon): It targets the sleep-wake cycle and does not depress the central nervous system as done by other drugs. Those having difficulty in falling asleep are prescribed this drug. It may be given for long term use.

4.		Silenor (Doxipine): It is recommended for people who have difficulty in staying asleep. It helps by blocking histamine receptors. Patient needs to sleep for seven to eight hours and dose should be carefully designed taking into consideration the age, health and response to therapy.

5.		Sonata (Zaleplon): It stays in the body for the shortest time as compared to other drugs. If the patient wakes up in midnight the dose may be repeated without feeling drowsy in the morning.

6.		Benzodiazepines: These are older drugs for insomnia and are prescribed when sleeplessness stays for long periods. They are effective in treating problems like sleep walking and night terrors. These drugs may cause drowsiness in the day time and may cause dependence that means you need to take the drug to be able to sleep.

7.	Antidepressants: These are effective in treating sleeplessness and anxiety.

Most of the pills have antihistamine as the primary active ingredient and are sold without prescription. Precaution must be taken if taking other drugs containing antihistamines like cold and allergy medications.

Q Can you find a good night's sleep at the drugstore?

Almost everyone suffers from trouble sleeping at one time or another. Insomnia—the inability to sleep—isn't a single disorder itself, but rather a general symptom like fever or pain.

Most of us experience disturbed sleep at some time or other, when late night we are awake or wake up early morning and are unable to sleep; turning sides in the bed, there may be many reasons for it. It may be a due to psychological or emotional issues, or mild depression. It may also be related to ageing. Sometimes when you do not find any reason for sleeplessness, which is technically known as insomnia. It may be for a short period or may prolong over weeks. People may feel drowsiness during day but are unable to nap, which may cause them to become forgetful and are not able to concentrate on the job. Underlying cause if it is properly treated, insomnia usually improves. If not improved, people go for sleeping pills.

Sleeping aids:

Nearly half of insomnia stems from underlying psychological or emotional issues. Stressful events, mild depression, or an anxiety disorder can keep people awake at night. When the underlying cause is properly treated, insomnia usually improves. If not, additional strategies to help promote sleep may be needed.

Lack of proper sleep can increase insulin resistance that increases the risk for the developing type 2 diabetes and heart problems. Shortened sleep can increase CRP, or C-reactive protein, which is released with stress and inflammation. "If your CRP is high, it's a risk factor for cardiovascular and heart disease".

SLEEP APNEA

It is a potentially serious sleep disorder in which breathing repeatedly stops and starts. If you snore loudly and feel tired even after a full night's sleep, you might have sleep apnea.

The main types of sleep apnea are:

•	Obstructive sleep apnea, the more common form that occurs when throat muscles relax

•	Central sleep apnea, which occurs when your brain doesn't send proper signals to the muscles that control breathing

•	Complex sleep apnea syndrome, also known as treatment-emergent central sleep apnea, which occurs when someone has both obstructive sleep apnea and central sleep apnea

Symptoms

•	Loud snoring

•	Episodes in which you stop breathing during sleep — which would be reported by another person

•	Gasping for air during sleep

•	Awakening with a dry mouth

•	Morning headache

•	Difficulty staying asleep (insomnia)

•	Excessive daytime sleepiness

•	Difficulty paying attention while awake

•	Irritability

CAUSES

Obstructive sleep apnea

This occurs when the muscles in the back of your throat relax. These muscles support the soft palate, the triangular piece of tissue hanging from the soft palate (uvula), the tonsils, the side walls of the throat and the tongue.

When the muscles relax, your airway narrows or closes as you breathe in. You can't get enough air, which can lower the oxygen level in your blood. Your brain senses your inability to breathe and briefly rouses you from sleep so that you can reopen your airway. This awakening is usually so brief that you don't remember it.

You might snort, choke or gasp. This pattern can repeat itself five to 30 times or more each hour, all night, impairing your ability to reach the deep, restful phases of sleep.

CENTRAL SLEEP APNEA

This less common form of sleep apnea occurs when your brain fails to transmit signals to your breathing muscles. This means that you make no effort to breathe for a short period. You might awaken with shortness of breath or have a difficult time getting to sleep or staying asleep.

Factors that increase the risk of sleep apnea include:

•	Excess weight. Obesity greatly increases the risk of sleep apnea. Fat deposits
	around your upper airway can obstruct your breathing.
•	Neck circumference. People with thicker necks might have narrower airways.

•	A narrowed airway. You might have inherited a narrow throat. Tonsils or
	adenoids also can enlarge and block the airway, particularly in children.
•	Being male. Men are two to three times more likely to have sleep apnea than
	are women. However, women increase their risk if they're overweight, and
	their risk also appears to rise after menopause.
•	Being older: Sleep apnea occurs significantly more often in older adults.

•	Family history: Having family members with sleep apnea might increase your
	risk.

•   Use of alcohol, sedatives or tranquilizers. These substances relax the muscles
in your throat, which can worsen obstructive sleep apnea.

•   Smoking. Smokers are three times more likely to have obstructive sleep
apnea than are people who've never smoked. Smoking can increase the
amount of inflammation and fluid retention in the upper airway.

•   Nasal congestion. If you have difficulty breathing through your nose —
whether from an anatomical problem or allergies — you're more likely to
develop obstructive sleep apnea.

Risk factors for this form of sleep apnea include:

•   Being older. Middle-aged and older people have a higher risk of central
sleep apnea.

•   Being male. Central sleep apnea is more common in men than it is in
women.

•   Heart disorders. Having congestive heart failure increases the risk.

•   Using narcotic pain medications. Opioid medications, especially long-
acting ones such as methadone, increase the risk of central sleep apnea.

•   Stroke. Having had a stroke increases your risk of central sleep apnea or
treatment-emergent central sleep apnea.

SLEEP APNEA AND HEART DISEASE

Sudden drops in blood oxygen levels that occur during sleep apnea increase blood pressure and strain the cardiovascular system. Having obstructive sleep apnea increases your risk of high blood pressure (hypertension).

Obstructive sleep apnea might also increase your risk of recurrent heart attack, stroke and abnormal heartbeats, such as atrial fibrillation. If you have heart disease, multiple episodes of low blood oxygen (hypoxia or hypoxemia) can lead to sudden death from an irregular heartbeat.

MENOPAUSAL HORMONE THERAPY

Long-term hormone replacement therapy used to be routinely prescribed for postmenopausal women to relieve hot flashes and other menopause symptoms. Hormone replacement therapy was also thought to reduce the risk of heart disease.

Before menopause, women have a lower risk of heart disease than men do. But as women age, and their oestrogen levels decline after menopause, their risk of heart disease increases. In the 1980s and 1990s, experts advised older women to take oestrogen and other hormones to keep their hearts healthy.

However, hormone replacement therapy — or menopause hormone therapy, as it's now called — has had mixed results. Many of the hoped-for benefits failed to materialize for large numbers of women. The largest randomized, controlled trial found a small increase in heart disease in postmenopausal women using combined (both oestrogen and progestin) hormone therapy. For women in this study using oestrogen alone, there was no increased risk in heart disease.

Risks in perspective

If you're having a tough time with symptoms of menopause but worry about how hormone therapy will affect your heart, consider these points:

• The risk of heart disease to an individual woman taking hormone therapy is very low. If you are in early menopause, have moderate to severe hot flashes and other menopausal symptoms, and are otherwise healthy, the benefits of hormone therapy likely outweigh any potential risks of heart disease.

•	Your individual risk of developing heart disease depends on many factors, including family medical history, personal medical history and lifestyle practices. Talk to your doctor about your personal risks. If you're at low risk of heart disease, and your menopausal symptoms are significant, hormone therapy is a reasonable consideration.

•	Risk differs for women with premature menopause or premature ovarian failure. If you stopped having periods before age 40 (premature menopause) or lost normal function of your ovaries before age 40 (premature ovarian failure), you have a different set of heart and blood vessel (cardiovascular) health risks compared with women who reach menopause near the average age of about 50. This includes a higher risk of coronary heart disease. If you have premature ovarian failure, you'll likely be given hormone therapy to protect against heart disease.

Menopause hormone therapy risks may vary depending on:

•	Whether oestrogen is given alone or with a progestin

•	Your current age and age at menopause

•	The dose, type of oestrogen and route, or how you take it (oral, transdermal,
	transvaginal)

•	Other health risks, such as your family medical history and cancer risks

WHO SHOULD NOT TAKE HORMONE THERAPY?

If you've already had a heart attack, menopause hormone therapy is not for you. If you already have heart disease or you have a history of blood clots, the risks of hormone therapy have been clearly shown to outweigh any potential benefits.

You can limit the risks:

•   Try a form of hormone therapy that has limited systemic effects. Estrogen and progestin are available in many forms, including pills, skin patches, gels, vaginal creams, and slow-releasing suppositories or rings that you place in your vagina. Low-dose vaginal preparations of estrogen — which come in cream, tablet or ring form — can effectively treat vaginal symptoms while minimizing absorption into the body. Similarly, hormones delivered through skin patches aren't as extensively metabolized in the body and have less potential for unwanted side effects.

•   Minimize the amount of medication you take. Use the lowest effective dose for the shortest amount of time needed to treat symptoms, unless you're younger than age 45 — in that case, you need enough estrogen for protection against long-term health effects of oestrogen deficiency. If you have lasting menopausal symptoms that significantly impair your quality of life, your doctor may recommend longer term treatment.

•	Make healthy lifestyle choices. Counter the risks of developing heart disease by making heart-healthy lifestyle choices. Don't smoke or use tobacco products. Get regular physical activity. Eat a healthy diet focusing on fruits, vegetables, whole grains and low-fat protein. Maintain a healthy weight and get regular health screenings to check your blood pressure and cholesterol levels to detect early signs of heart disease.

•	Seek regular follow-up care. See your health care provider regularly to ensure that the benefits of hormone therapy continue to outweigh the risks, and for cancer screenings such as mammograms and pelvic exams.

COOKING OILS

A variety of cooking oils are available in the market. It is very difficult to determine which should be preferred for a safe heart. In different parts of the world different oils are in use depending upon the availability of the raw material. In Gujarat peanut oil is mostly used while in Kerala coconut oil is preferred. In central India mustard oil is more common. In fact, healthy cooking oil is that which contains more of polyunsaturated fatty acids (PUFA).

What does the term "saturated or polyunsaturated oil" mean?

Chemically, oil is made up of chains of carbon, hydrogen and oxygen called fatty acids. All fatty acids consist a chain of carbon atoms with varying amounts of hydrogen atoms attached to them. A molecule that has two hydrogen atoms attached to each carbon atom is said to be saturated, because it is holding all the hydrogen atoms it possibly can. A fatty acid which is missing a pair of hydrogen atoms on one of its carbon is called monounsaturated fat. If more than two hydrogen atoms are missing, it is called polyunsaturated fat.

WHAT ARE OMEGA-3 AND OMEGA-6 FATTY ACIDS?

These fatty acids are considered to be essential for human beings. They are important structural components of the cell membrane and serve as substrate for the synthesis of a variety of potent hormones collectively known as Prostaglandins. These essential fatty acids may form different types of prostaglandins which may have different physiological functions. In the diet of modern American societies, the ratio of Omega-6 to Omega-3 is 10:3 while in the diet of the primitive man this ratio was much low. There are three principal types of Omega-3 fatty acids. They are

(1)   Alpha-linolenic acid (ALA), (2) Eicosapentaenoic acid (EPA) and Docosahexaenoic acid (DHA). ALA is found in large amount in flaxseed and its oil. Also, it is found in small amount in canola and soy bean oils. EPA and DHA are found mainly in sea food and in some cold-water fatty fishes like herring, mackerel, salmon and sardines. In varying amounts, they are also found in algae and other aquatic plants. Most fresh water fishes have less omega-3 fatty acids than fatty salt water fishes. Fresh water trout however has high levels of omega-3 fatty acids. Fishes like Tilapia and Catfish are not heart healthy as they have high levels of unhealthy fatty acids. Also, it is important how the fish is cooked. It is better to consume baked fish and not the deep fried. Human body is capable of converting ALA into EPA and DHA.

These fatty acids when substituted by saturated fatty acids such as those of meat may lower cholesterol level in the blood.

Omega-3s particularly EPA and DHA from fish oil help in protecting the heart as they have moderate capability to reduce blood pressure and improve blood lipids. Omega 3s from fish or fish oil decrease serum Triglycerides and VLDLs (very low-density lipoproteins) levels by 30% or more. It increases HDL-C level in those who have high Triglyceride level (>200mg/dl). Consumption of two servings of fish per week is able to reduce by 40% the risk of dying with cardiovascular disease. Omega effects inhibit the production of thromboxane A2 (Tx A2) and inflammatory cytokines. Both of these have tendency to check the clotting of blood which is the major cause of heart attack. In those who are taking aspirin to reduce blood clotting, consumption of Omega-3s attenuates the effect of aspirin. In some patients the heart rate becomes arrhythmic. Omega-3s has antiarrhythmic property. Supplementation of Omega-3s is recommended in their diet

Omega-6 fatty acids are in large amounts in grains.

The high proportion of oxidation prone linolenic acid is undesirable in cooking oils. Unsaturated fatty acids are necessary for our body, however, during cooking they are transformed into trans-fats which are very harmful. Snacks available in the market have good amount of trans - fats as they are fried in hydrogenated vegetable oils manufactured to make the food last longer. It is recommended that oil once used for frying should not be used again because during second cooking when the temperature reaches its smoking point it rapidly changes into Trans –fat.

Hydrogenated vegetable oils contain high proportion of trans-fatty acids. Medical research suggests that high ratio of omega-6 fatty acids and omega-3 fatty acids may increase the probability of a number of diseases and depression. The optimal ratio should be 4:1 or lower. A high intake of omega-6 fatty acids may increase the risk of breast cancer in postmenopausal women and of prostate cancer in men.

MUSTERED OIL

Extracted from mustered (*Brassica nigra*) seeds it is largely used as cooking oil in Northern and Eastern India. It has pungent aroma due to Allyl isothiocynate. Composition is given in Table: It is cheap and is a good source of high omega-3 fatty acids. In Indian culinary mustered oil is heated to smoking before cooking to reduce its strong smell and taste. However, high heat can damage the omega-3 fatty acids in the oil reducing its health benefits.

It is recently reported that in the regions where mustered oil is traditionally being used for cooking it may afford some protection against cardiovascular diseases. It is true only when fresh oil is used in small quantities. It is possible that its effect is due to uric acid to make blood platelets less sticky or due to the presence of high percentage of alpha-linolenic acid. The exact mode of action is not known.

OLIVE OIL

It is extracted from olive - the fruit of *Olea europaea* which is a traditional tree crop of mediterrerian countries like Spain, Italy and Greece. The oil is obtained by whole olives and extracting the oil by mechanical or chemical methods. It is largely used in cooking, cosmetics, medicine, and has many other applications. The grades of the oil extracted from olive fruit can be classified as:

1.   Virgin or extra virgin olive oil—Oil produced by the use of physical means only and no chemicals are used for extraction.

2.   Refined olive oil—Oil that has been chemically treated to suppress the unwanted taste and fatty acids. This is commonly regarded as oil of lower quality than virgin oil

3.   Olive Pomace oil   - It is the oil extracted from pomace using solvents and by heat.

Beside these three principal grades, several types of olive oils are available in the market depending on their acid content and are blended with refined oil. Olive oil is mainly composed of mixed triglyceride esters of oleic acid and palmitic acid and of other fatty acids and antioxidants like vitamin E and carotenoids that may help in preventing oxidation of LDL particles. Details of composition of olive oil are given in Table below.

As they are least processed forms of olive oil extra virgin or virgin oil have more monosaturated fatty acids than other olive oils. These types also have more polyphenols, which are beneficial for the heart. Olive oil contains valuable antioxidants that are not found in other oils. They are believed to have a protective effect against certain cancers and peptic ulcers.

Extra virgin olive oil is used mostly as a salad dressing and with food to be eaten cold. When extra virgin olive oil is heated to 170 C the unrefined particles burn and that deteriorates the taste. For those who heat the oil to a high temperature it is recommended to use refined olive oil for frying and should be replaced after several uses. One tbsp i.e., 13.5-gram olive oil contains following nutritional components.

Calories: 119

Fat: 13.50

Carbohydrates: 0

Fiber: 0

Protein: 0

Significantly high content of monosaturated fatty acids (72%) makes it the first choice among edible oil for reduction in the risk of coronary heart disease. It is also credited to lower blood cholesterol, anti-inflammatory, antihypertensive as well as for vasodilatory and HDL raising effects. It also displaces omega-6 fatty acids while there is no effect on omega-3 fatty acids.

PEANUT OIL

Extracted from ground nut (*Arachis hypogea*) it is popular cooking oil as it is inexpensive and relatively low in saturated fats. From highly refined oil all the allergens are removed. It performs quite good at high temperature also, hence is used for deep frying; however, it has a slight nutty flavor which suits many a cuisine.

COCONUT OIL

It is extracted from mature coconuts (*Coco nucifera*). It is very commonly used in Southern India and Ceylon for preparation of various dishes but it has high level of saturated fatty acids which makes it less appealing to those who are careful about fatty acid consumption. Coconut oil has lowest cholesterol content.

SOYBEAN OIL

It is extracted from the seeds of soybean (*Glycine max*) and is widely used in cooking. It has both the major monounsaturated fatty acids and saturated fatty acids. The major unsaturated fatty acids in soybean are triglycerides, alpha-linolenic acid, linoleic acid and oleic acid. It also has saturated fatty acids stearic acid and palmic acid.

PALM OIL

It is extracted from the mesocarp of the fruit of the oil palm (*Eaelis guineensis*). It is different from palm kernel oil. It does not contain the red pigment. It is 14 % saturated while palm kernel oil is 81 % saturated. It is semisolid at room temperature and contains many saturated and unsaturated fats. Like all vegetable oils palm oil contains very little cholesterol, although it increases both LDL and HDL cholesterol. It is low in cost and its refined product has high oxidative stability making it favored oil for frying.

The approximate concentration of fatty acids in palm oil is:

TYPE OF FATTY ACID%

Myristic saturated C14	1, 0
Palmitic saturated C16	43.5
Stearic saturated C18	4.3
Oleic monosaturated C18	36.6
Linoleic acid C18	9.1
Others	5.5

CORN OIL

It is extracted from the germ of maize (*Zea maize*). Its refined product is valuable frying oil. It is also largely used in margarines as it is comparatively cheaper.

SESAME OIL

It is extracted from Sesame (*Sesamum indicum*) seeds and is commonly used in Chinese dishes as it has a rich nutty aroma and is rich in antioxidants.

FLAXSEED OIL

It is extracted from Linseed (*Linum usitatissimum*) not good for cooking but it is healthy if used in garnishing when used raw as it contains all the goodness of omega-3 and omega-6. Its low smoke point categorizes it as delicate oil which has to be stored in refrigerator. This oil has a slightly bitter taste but it is masked by the food it is served with. Mostly used in salad dressings.

WALNUT OIL

Extracted from walnut (*Jinglans regia*), it is an important component of mediterrarian cuisine. It has antioxidant properties. Since its smoke point is not very high it can be used in cooking at medium temperature.

BUTTER

It is used in wide verities of dishes, on the breakfast table and largely in confectionary. A Swedish study showed that consumption of butter reduces fat level in blood. This may be because butter has short and medium fatty acid chains as compared to those of vegetable oils. It is also considered to be preferred by the human digestive system. It may also be usefully added to the low fat foods such as vegetables to lower the feeling of hunger. People with milk allergies should avoid butter which contains enough of allergy causing proteins to cause reactions.

FREQUENTLY ASKED QUESTIONS

Q. How much oil should be used by an individual?

A. Amount of oil to be used depends upon age, sex and type of body work of the individual. If somebody is consuming 1400 calories in one day, 280 may come from oils. Women between 19-30 years taking regular exercise of half an hour can consume six table spoons of oil. Those above 30 should take oil not more than 5 table spoons. Males (19-30 years) can take seven table spoons of oil while those above 30 years should not take more than six table spoons.

Q. Which oil should be used for cooking?

A. It is not good to always use the same oil because different oils have different properties. Flex oil has more vitamin B while sunflower oil does not have bad cholesterol. Some oils are capable of countering the heart ailment while others are full of nutrients. Our body requires all these things. Omega3 and omega6 are not made by our body, therefore we require them. Doctors therefore recommend that the oil should be changed after 2-3 months selecting only good quality oils. It is better to use oil which does not stick to the utensil after cooking.

Q. How to store the cooking oils?

A. If oils are exposed to open air and sunlight, their unsaturated fatty acids are oxidized and become harmful. Sunflower and peanut oils are more reactive. Therefore, they should be kept in tightly closed containers for about six months. Olive oil may be kept for about one year.

Properties of different cooking oils (Serving size 14 grams)					
	Calor-ies	Unsat-urated fat (Gram)	Satur-ated fat (gram)	Smoke point (°C)	
Peanut oil	120	10.5	1.5	232	
Coconut oil	117	1.8	11.8	350	
Walnut oil	120	12	2.0	160	
Avocado oil	120	12	2.0	271	
Sesame oil	120	11	1.9	232	
Flaxseed oil	120	11,2	1.3	107	

Coconut oil has been used throughout Asia and the Pacific for thousands of years as both a food and a medicine.
Even today it holds a highly respected position in the Ayurvedic medicine of India. Only recently has modern medical research confirmed the many health benefits traditionally attributed to this remarkable oil.

Once mistakenly thought to be bad because of its saturated fat content, coconut oil is now known to contain a unique form of saturated fat that actually helps prevent heart disease, stroke, and hardening of the arteries. The saturated fat in coconut oil is unlike the fat found in meat or other vegetable fats. It is identical to a special group of fats found in human breast milk which have been shown to improve digestion, strengthen the immune system, and protect against bacterial, viral, and fungal infections.

These fats, derived from coconut oil, are now routinely used in hospital IV formulations and commercial baby formulas. They're also used in sports drinks to boost energy and enhance athletic performance.

Some of the benefits of coconut oil:
- Reduces risk of atherosclerosis and related illnesses
- Reduces risk of cancer and other degenerative conditions
- Helps prevent bacterial, viral, and fungal (including yeast) infections
- Supports immune system function
- Helps prevent osteoporosis
- Helps control diabetes
- Promotes weight loss
- Supports healthy metabolic function
- Provides an immediate source of energy
- Supplies fewer calories than other fats
- Supplies important nutrients necessary for good health
- Improves digestion and nutrient absorption
- Is highly resistant to spoilage (long shelf life)
- Is heat resistant (the healthiest oil for cooking)
- Helps keep skin soft and smooth
- Helps prevent premature aging and wrinkling of the skin

·   Helps protect against skin cancer and other blemishes

Coconut oil has been called the "healthiest dietary oil on earth." If you're not using coconut oil for your daily cooking and body care needs, you're missing out on one of nature's most amazing health products.

NITRIC OXIDE

Nitric oxide is vital for a healthy cardiovascular system, but deep breathing is just a start. Produced by the endothelium—the lining of the blood vessels—this chemical is highly responsive to healthy heart habits like regular exercise and low cholesterol. Lowering cholesterol levels helps increase nitric oxide. These lifestyle measures turn the nitric oxide spigots on, expanding blood vessels and increasing blood flow while curbing the build-up of plaque. (Nitric oxide is the basis for the use of nitro-glycerine in treating the heart condition, angina.)

The opposite is true, however. When heart disease risk factors like smoking, a poor diet, lack of exercise and even psychological distress are present, levels of nitric oxide plummet and blood vessels begin to accumulate fatty plaque, setting the stage for atherosclerosis. Heart attack or stroke can occur if the plaque becomes inflamed and ruptures.

The keys to raising nitric oxide are mentioned below:

•	Eat right. Fill your plate with fruits and vegetables, lean protein and whole grains, and limit your intake of fat, sugar and salt.

•	Get moving. Incorporate regular activity into your life and try to achieve and maintain a healthy weight.

•	Lower risk factors. Aim to normalize your blood pressure, cholesterol, and blood sugar levels, using medications, if needed and prescribed by your doctor.

•	Finally, don't forget to breathe! Slowly now, through your nose for a few minutes, especially if you're feeling stressed.

HARDENING OF ARTERIES (ARTERIOSCLEROSIS)

Blood vessels of various sizes form the peripheral circulation in the form of long channels and networks to distribute nutrition and oxygen to billions of cells of our body. Blood vessels are of three types:

1.   **Arteries**: These are thick walled and elastic which carry the blood away from the heart. The wall of the artery has three layers. The outermost is tunica adventitia which firmly supports the wall. The middle layer is tunica media which has thick muscular layer. The innermost is the tunica intima which forms the inner lining of the vessel and is in contact with the blood. The largest arterial blood vessel is the aorta which arises from the left ventricle. It ramifies into smaller vessels which further ramify into finer arteries known as arterioles and end up in capillaries which distribute blood to the various organs.

2.   **Veins**: They are thin-walled elastic blood vessels which collect impure blood from the tissues and take it to the heart. They also have three layers but they are quite thin.

3.   **Capillaries**: They are very thin blood vessels which connect the arteries and veins. Through these capillaries the nutrients and oxygen are transferred to the tissues and from the tissues waste material is collected.

Hardening of the arteries is not a disease of modern civilization as is generally believed. It has been described in 3500 years old mummies excavated after centuries of burial. Arteriosclerosis is the cause of disease and death as it involves coronary and cerebral arteries resulting in coronary artery disease, cerebral thrombosis and apoplectic strokes. With the onset of disease, the arteries may be affected and may lead to clinical complications. Blood flow may be blocked depriving organs like heart or brain of oxygen and nutrients. Hardening of the artery is commonly termed as arteriosclerosis. Mostly middle coat of the artery is affected but it is rather harmless, however, when inner layer or tunica intima is affected, it may lead to physiological complications.

Three main types of arteriosclerosis are described.

1.   **Monck Berg's sclerosis**: In this case calcium deposits in the middle layer as a result of which the arteries become beaded or whip like mostly in the arms, and legs of elderly people. This type of hardening is not harmful.

2.   **Atherosclerosis**: Large or medium size arteries are affected namely the aorta, coronary arteries and the arteries supplying the brain. In this case there is deposition of fats, blood clots, calcium and fibrous tissue in the inner coat of the artery. This development or atheroma blocks or restricts the free supply of blood to the organ concerned.

3.   **Arteriosclerosis**: In this type small vessels of the kidney and other vital organs show an overgrowth on the inner wall. This is usually associated with high blood pressure.

Atherosclerosis is responsible for more deaths than any other disease. 95 percent of heart patients die due to coronary disease and 50 percent brain deaths are due to diseases of the brain vessels. It has been regarded for long that hardening of the arteries is incurable and is a disease associated with age. It has now been realized that it is not true as people more than 70 or 80 years have been shown at autopsy* to be free of coronary disease while several cases are now on record which tell about increasing population of young coronary artery disease patients. Young adults with congenital or rheumatic heart show severe hardening of the pulmonary arteries. It is now believed that arteriosclerosis is a metabolic disease with excessive amount of cholesterol in the circulating blood. Causative factors involved in atherosclerosis are as yet not very clear. There is a relationship between fats in the diet, cholesterol level and formation of atheroma.

Now a day there is emphasis on the quality of fats ingested than on the quantity ingested. Opinion today says that ingestion of high quantities of animal fats and saturated fatty acids play important role in the onset of atherosclerosis and that consumption of unsaturated fatty acids may not only serve to replace saturated fatty acids but may also neutralize to some extent their ill effects. Heredity, body build, sex, race, age and diseases like diabetes and high blood pressure are also important causative factors.

* Post-mortem examination to discover the extent of disease/cause of death.

Dietary modifications may play great role in restricting the consumption of animal fat and supplementation of unsaturated fatty acids such as sunflower and soybean oil may be added to the meals. Foods may be baked, boiled, broiled, steamed or roasted but not fried.

Physical exercise and avoiding smoking help a lot in maintaining the health of the arteries.

TREATMENT OF HEART DISEASE

INTERVENTIONS

1.   CPR Cardiopulmonary resuscitation - CPR. Learn CPR for a loved one.

2.   Stents- Get information about why they're used and what types are   available.

3.   Angioplasty and Stents Angioplasty is a procedure that uses very little   cutting to open blocked heart arteries. Stents can be put in during angioplasty.

4.   Heart Bypass Surgery: This can treat heart disease when your coronary   arteries are blocked. Your doctor may treat the problem by giving the blood a new pathway to the heart.

5.   Valve Disease Treatment: When your heart valve disease needs attention; it can be treated by traditional surgery or by balloon valvuloplasty, which doesn't require as much cutting.

6.   Cardioversion: For many people with heart disease, drugs alone won't turn an arrhythmia into a normal heart rhythm. These people may need a procedure called cardioversion or electrical cardioversion.

7.   EECP: This can help stimulate blood vessels to develop small branches, creating a natural bypass around narrowed or blocked arteries that cause chest pain.

8.   Pacemaker: It's a small device that sends electrical impulses to the heart muscle to keep up a suitable heart rate and rhythm. A pacemaker may also treat fainting spells (syncope), congestive heart failure, and hypertrophic cardiomyopathy.

9.   Implantable Cardioverter Defibrillators (ICD): An ICD, or implantable cardioverter defibrillator, can treat abnormal heart rhythms.

10.   Lead Extraction: That's removal of one or more leads from inside the heart. Leads that are placed outside the heart during open heart surgery cannot be removed by this procedure.

11.   Left Ventricular Assist Device (LVAD): It's a kind of mechanical heart. A surgeon would place it inside your chest. It would help the heart pump oxygen-rich blood throughout the body.

12.   Heart Transplant: A person's diseased heart is replaced with a healthy donor's heart. The donor is a person who has died and whose family has agreed to donate their loved one's organs.

MEDICATIONS

13.   ACE Inhibitors: Angiotensin converting enzyme (ACE) inhibitors are heart meds that widen, or dilate, your blood vessels to raise the amount of blood your heart pumps and lower your blood pressure.

14.   Angiotensin II Receptor Blockers: These heart drugs decrease certain chemicals that narrow blood vessels. This allows blood to flow more easily throughout your body. These drugs also decrease chemicals that cause salt and fluid to build up in the body.

15.   Antiarrhythmic Drugs: These drugs treat abnormal heart rhythms caused by irregular electrical activity of your heart.

16.   Antiplatelet Drugs: They are a group of powerful medications that prevent the formation of blood clots.

17.   Aspirin Therapy: For more than 100 years, aspirin has been used as a pain reliever. Since the 1970s, aspirin has also been used to prevent and manage heart disease and stroke.

18.   Beta-Blocker Therapy: Beta-blocker is one of the most widely prescribed classes of drugs to treat hypertension (high blood pressure). They are a mainstay treatment for congestive heart failure.

19.   Calcium Channel Blocker Drugs: These relax blood vessels and increase the supply of blood and oxygen to the heart. They also reduce the heart's workload.

20.   Clot Buster Drugs: Also called thrombolytic therapy, these are a type of heart medication given in the hospital through the veins (intravenous) to break up blood clots.

21.   Digoxin: If you have heart disease, this is a medicine that helps an injured or weakened heart work more efficiently.

22.   Diuretics: You may hear these called water pills. They help your body get rid of unneeded water and salt through urine. That makes it easier for your heart to pump. It also helps control your blood pressure.

23.   Nitrates: These are meds that treat angina in people with coronary artery disease. They also help ease chest pain caused by blocked blood vessels of the heart.

24.   Warfarin and Other Blood Thinners: These medicines help prevent clots from forming. Blood thinners treat some types of heart disease.

CARE

25.   Plant-Based Diet for Heart Health: Early studies suggests it may have a number of benefits.

26.   Recovery after Heart Surgery: There are things you should know when you or someone you love comes back from heart surgery.

27.   Finding Strength during Tough Times: Caregivers should be mindful of the psychological, social, cultural, and spiritual aspects of health and illness, as well as the effects of these factors on themselves and their loved ones.

WARNING SIGNS OF HEART ATTACK

Common heart attack signs and symptoms include:

•   Pressure, tightness, pain, or a squeezing or aching sensation in your chest or arms that may spread to your neck, jaw or back

•   Nausea, indigestion, heartburn or abdominal pain

•   Shortness of breath

•   Cold sweat

•   Fatigue

•   Light headedness or sudden dizziness

Heart attack symptoms may vary

Not all people who have heart attacks have the same symptoms or have the same severity of symptoms. Some people have mild pain; others have more severe pain. Some people have no symptoms; for others, the first sign may be of sudden cardiac arrest. However, the more signs and symptoms you have, the greater the likelihood you're having a heart attack.

Some heart attacks strike suddenly, but many people have warning signs and symptoms hours, days or weeks in advance. The earliest warning might be recurrent chest pain or pressure (angina) that's triggered by exertion and relieved by rest. Angina is caused by a temporary decrease in blood flow to the heart.

Get help quickly

Act immediately. Some people wait too long because they don't recognize the important signs and symptoms. Take these steps:

•	Call for emergency medical help. If you suspect you're having a heart attack, don't hesitate. Immediately call ambulance or your local emergency number. If you don't have access to emergency medical services, have someone drive you to the nearest hospital.

Drive yourself only if there are no other options. Because your condition can worsen, driving yourself puts you and others at risk.

•	Take nitro-glycerine, if prescribed to you by a doctor. Take it as instructed while awaiting emergency help.

•	Take aspirin, if recommended. Taking aspirin during a heart attack could reduce heart damage by helping to keep your blood from clotting.

Aspirin can interact with other medications, however, so don't take an aspirin unless your doctor or emergency medical personnel recommend it. Don't delay. Call for emergency help first.

What to do if you see someone who might be having a heart attack?

If you see someone who's unconscious and you believe is having a heart attack, first call for emergency medical help. Then check if the person is breathing and has a pulse. If the person isn't breathing or you don't find a pulse, only then you should begin CPR to keep blood flowing.

Push hard and fast on the person's chest in a fairly rapid rhythm — about 100 to 120 compressions a minute.

If you haven't been trained in CPR, doctors recommend performing only chest compressions. If you have been trained in CPR, you can go on to opening the airway and rescue breathing.

Recovery is usually determined by how severe the heart attack is. In the simplest cases, only one coronary vessel is blocked, and it is treated quickly so there's minimal damage to the heart muscle. If the heart function is normal, those patients can really be discharged from the hospital pretty quickly. When there is more damage, either because the patient doesn't get to the hospital quickly enough or because there are more arteries involved, it's more complicated. In these cases, the patient will normally stay in the hospital longer as we're assessing heart function and identifying the right medication to help heal the heart.

The most severe level occurs when the patient has multiple blockages and needs bypass surgery. In that case, the hospitalization and recovery are going to be much more complicated.

WHEN YOU LEAVE THE HOSPITAL.......

It is important for MI survivors to complete inpatient and out-patient cardiac rehab. Cardiac rehab has been shown to lower mortality in patients who have a heart attack. If patient is in pretty good health, it is encouraged to start as soon as possible. Patients who have bypass surgery start within the first couple of weeks after surgery.

After rehab, being physically active most days of the week is essential. If you need to lower your cholesterol or blood pressure, aim for 40 minutes of moderate-to-vigorous physical activity three to four times per week.

Medication is an important part of post-MI treatment. MI survivors should also take a baby aspirin every day, and if they've had a stent, they need an additional anticoagulant or antiplatelet medication to prevent clots from forming within the stent.

Because most survivors have high blood pressure, they will usually be on at least one medication to control it. But even without hypertension, after a MI, medications that lower blood pressure, such as ACEI and beta blockers, may be recommended due to the damage to the heart.

AVOIDING ANOTHER MI AND READMISSION

Nobody wants a second MI or another hospital stay, but about 18 percent of survivors are readmitted. Survivors can certainly improve their chances of recovery and avoid readmissions by taking the recommended actions of their medical team seriously and sticking to them.

An important step is to make — and keep — a follow up appointment with the cardiologist.

Patients should come to their follow-up appointments armed with questions. Talk about any symptoms they are having so the doctor can either reassure them it's nothing serious, or so the doctor can be aware of the situation and monitor it. Are there any side effects from medications? Anticoagulants and anti-platelet drugs can cause bleeding, and blood in the stool can be a symptom. Is there increased shortness of breath and swelling in the ankles?

When you get home from the hospital after cardiac surgery you are not normal physically and mentally. You are not able to do certain things; therefore, it is necessary that you apply check on your wishes. This condition will persist for a short duration in order to give your body a chance to heal. Following account discusses some of the important points

- **Walk**: Take complete sleep. Get up by 7 A.M. Have a cup of tea and go for a small walk initially. Every week add five minutes to your walk till it is 25 to 30 minutes. After breakfast take a nap. Read newspaper. Before lunch have a small walk. After lunch go to sleep for 1 to 2 hours. In the evening also go for a walk.

• **Diet**: You should eat a low salt, low cholesterol diet to keep your heart healthy. If you are diabetic, you should continue the prescribed diet. You may not have much appetite but it is important to eat as your body needs nourishment for healing. Follow the hand out given by the hospital to see what food you should and should not eat.

• **Pain**: After surgery there is some muscle or incision discomfort. You may feel tightness or numbness along the incision but it should not be similar to what you experienced before the surgery. You shall be given prescription for pain. If saphenous vein from your leg has been used for graft, toughness will be felt for some weeks. Over the time discomfort and stiffness will go.

• **Driving**: Do not drive a car or scooter until your cardiologist allows. Up to four weeks avoid using a car. After this period, you may travel in the car but do not try to drive. You may be allowed to drive after 6 to 8 weeks, if your surgery was minimal invasive. Scooter/Bike should not be driven for at least four months, that too after the permission of the cardiologist.

• **Lifting**: Since you have incisions on your chest, it's important to take care of them for about four weeks- the time required for healing. Up to four weeks do not try to lift, pull or push anything heavier than 3 to 4 kilos. By this time, you shall be going to nearby market, but do not lift grocery bags or children. Do not play or swim without the permission of the doctor. Take care of your stitches as any infection may lead to hospitalization.

• **Resuming work**: House hold chores can be done, but standing in one place for more than 15 minutes is not recommended.

• **Gradually increase activity**: Most cardiac patients resume working sometime after surgery. The amount of time depends on the type of surgery you had, how quickly you heal and the type of work you do. Your cardiologist will tell you when to resume work. It may take time to go back to your regular activities so it is better to resume normal activity gradually. Keep a record of your body weight. Make sure you use the same scale and wear the same type of clothing every time. If you lose or gain more than two kilos in three days, just call upon your cardiologist.

•   **Smoking**: Do not smoke. Smoking increases your risk of hardening of blood vessels. If your willpower is not strong enough, you should contact organizations which help in quitting smoking.

•   **Emotions**: It is common to feel depressed and prone to anger after heart surgery. There are both physiological and psychological reasons for it. Depression and anger affect people differently. You may lose your appetite and lose the energy and desire to do much. All these symptoms go away gradually over few weeks. Engage yourself in talking to your dear ones and watching TV. Sometimes you may feel bad, sometimes good. It is better not to think about your illness and surgery, instead concentrate on your healing and getting back to normal life.

It is important that you tell all the doctors you consult that you had cardiac surgery. He may contact your cardiologist, if need be. You are not free to go for non-emergency procedures including dental cleaning up to six months after cardiac surgery without permission from the cardiologist. If you develop fever or sore throat, contact your cardiologist or physician.

You are required to see your cardiac surgeon 2 to 3 weeks after you leave the hospital.

You should call your surgeon immediately if:

☐   You have fever of 100.4^0 F.

☐   You see redness, swelling, yellow bad smelling drainage or opening of incision.

☐   Your pain killer is not effective.
☐   You have very tired feeling that will not go away even with rest.
☐   You find difficulty in breathing.
☐   You have persistent cough.
☐   You have swelling of your feet, ankles or legs.
☐   You have any unusual symptom.

Go to closest emergency clinic if:

- You have angina like chest pain or discomfort.
- Your heart is beating very fast (more than 150 beats per minute)
- You have irregular heartbeat.
- You feel shortness of breath that does not go with rest.
- Sudden weakness or numbness in arms or legs.
- Sudden severe headache.
- You faint.
- You cough up bright red blood.
- You see bright red blood in stool.

HEART DISEASE IN WOMEN

It was believed that only men have heart disease and women at risk only in older age. Recent studies show that about 1.3 million women have heart disease and their number increases every year. It is no more a disease of old age as 20% women under 65 years of age have heart attack each year. Also, the rate of heart disease in men is declining but that in women is at rise. Still only 25% women recognize heart disease as a big cause of death world over. The British Heart Foundation highlighted in its report that only 12 % women are aware of the most important factors responsible for heart attack. The causes of heart ailment also show some differences from men. Type II diabetes increases the risk in women than in men. Women smokers are at higher risk than men. Depression is also a more important factor for heart disease in women than in men. Women taking contraceptive pills are a risk three times than in men. In some women blood pressure rises during pregnancy, but at the time of delivery it drops. Such women may have high blood pressure later in life.

FREQUENTLY ASKED QUESTIONS

Q.   Do women show different signs for heart attack?

A study of National Institute of health (NIH) shows that women often experience new or different physical symptoms a month or more before experiencing heart attack. Among the 515 women studied 95% said they knew their symptoms were new or different quite before experiencing a heart attack. Women's symptoms are not as predictable as those of men.

Most women know the symptoms of a heart attack -- squeezing chest pain, shortness of breath and, nausea. But as it turns out, these symptoms are more typical for males. Female heart attacks can be quite different -- and it's important for all women to learn the warning signs.

Rhonda Monroe's story is a cautionary tale. She was mystified when strong pain struck her left breast and left arm. Monroe, who was a 36-year-old mother of three, didn't know it at the time, but she was having early symptoms of a heart attack. "I certainly wasn't thinking about my heart because I was young and healthy and had been skinny," she says. As the pain moved into her shoulder and back, Monroe took pain relievers. But the next day, she had nausea, sweating, vomiting, and chest pain. An ambulance rushed her to the emergency room.

Her next hurdle: getting the doctors to believe her. "They didn't take me seriously," Monroe says. She didn't fit the profile of a heart attack patient. The doctors told her she was too young, she was not overweight, and there was no family history of heart disease.

Frustrated by worsening pain and weakness Monroe returned to the hospital several times over the days that followed, only to come home with no answers.

Monroe turned to her primary care doctor about her situation and went through more tests at the hospital. Finally, she got her diagnosis -- a week after the initial breast and arm pain. As Monroe recalls, a cardiologist who had previously dismissed her complaints made the diagnosis. "The doctor told me, 'Well, it's a good thing you're persistent because you're having a heart attack."

Heart experts say Monroe's situation is all too common. Women who have "atypical" symptoms, such as arm or back pain or nausea, might not realize at first that they're having a heart attack. Then when they do seek emergency care, doctors sometimes misdiagnose them.

Q.   Is hormone replacement therapy useful for protecting the women from heart attack?

A.   Till few years ago the doctors had been giving hormonal replacement therapy to menopausal women considering estrogen and progesterone as heart protectors. But a 2002 US study showed that it did not protect the heart, rather it increased the risk of clotting. A trial of 16000 women was abandoned because many women showed evidence of an increased risk of breast cancer, stroke and heart disease. Also, the rate of heart disease and stroke was raised. It was suggested that they should take drug therapy and adopt dietary changes. However, women experiencing menopausal changes like hot flushes are still prescribed hormone replacement therapy. They are advised to have regular mammograms, pap smears and ultrasound to timely diagnosis of any adverse effects of hormone replacement therapy. It however, reduces chances of colorectal cancer and improves bone density.

Q. How does one know if her symptoms are serious?

A.   It is better to make it a habit to note typical aches and pains and normal reactions to foods and activities. This may help in recognizing when something is wrong. If she has a risk factor like high blood pressure, high cholesterol, diabetes or sedentary lifestyle, she should be especially careful about monitoring how she feels or she has any early signs of heart attack. If she feels worried or has unusual changes in her energy levels, comfort or sleep, she should discuss with the doctor.

Major symptoms prior to heart attack in women include:

- Unusual fatigue -70%
- Sleep disturbance—48%
- Shortness of breath—42%
- Indigestion—39%
- Anxiety—35%

Major symptoms during the heart attack include:

- Shortness of breath—58%
- Weakness in arms—55%
- Unusual fatigue—43%
- Cold sweat—39%
- Dizziness—39%

Some women may have heart attack without chest pain.

Q.   Is there any relation between heart disease and exercise in women?

A.   A study made on 74000 ethnically diverse post – menopausal women showed that those who walked for 30 minutes every day had lower risk of suffering a heart attack. Other studies have also confirmed this observation. It is therefore, very important to be physically active.

Q.   How does one know if her symptoms are serious?

A.   It is better to make it a habit to note typical aches and pains and normal reactions to foods and activities. This may help in recognizing when something is wrong. If she has a risk factor like high blood pressure, high cholesterol, diabetes or sedentary lifestyle, she should be especially careful about monitoring how she feels or she has any early signs of heart attack. If she feels worried or has unusual changes in her energy levels, comfort or sleep, she should discuss with the doctor.

Q.   Is there any relationship between lycopene and heart disease in women?

A.   Lycopene is a constituent of tomato juice. It is helpful in many diseases. Study on ischemic heart risk factors shows that lower serum lycopene in women is associated with risk of heart attack and stroke. Dr Sesso has reported in the journal of nutrition that Women with high intake of lycopene rich tomato-based food had a reduced risk of cardiovascular disease compared to women with low intake of these foods. Women having high level of lycopene (21.0 microgram /dl) also have high values of other beneficial carotenoids such as lutein, Zeaxanthin and alpha and beta carotene.

ROLE OF FAMILY IN PATIENT CARE

Family is a great asset for the patient of heart disease. It is always helpful to depute an adult family member for the care of the patient. The family should notice any changes that may occur in behavioral pattern of the patient. He may show depression, less interest in diet and recreation. His sleep pattern should also be noticed. The attendant and other members of the family should have frequent interaction with the patient. In the busy life of today, one hardly finds any time for others, but it is important that some time is shared with the patient. If he insists for normal food, he should be convinced to control his desires for a few days and should be told about the food prescribed by the doctor. Drugs should be administered at proper time. Entertainment is a vital factor in recouping. Family members can play cards with the patient and can read news for him. Television programs of his choice should be played. One family member should accompany him on walks. If the patient is depressed, every effort should be made to motivate him by diffusing his thinking about the illness. He should be pursued to take prescribed exercise. This will help in mood lifting. Utmost important is the love and affection to the patient. Visitors should not be allowed to sit long.

Environment also plays a great role in recoupment from the disease. The patient should be kept in a clean and well-ventilated room which is not very much isolated and at the same time not much crowded and disturbed. It is better to place the bed of the patient from where he can see outside view, particularly the trees. Alternatively, some flower pots may be put in the window. A wall clock and a call bell are must. The button of the call bell should be very much in the approach of the patient and the bell call should be attended promptly. Walls of the room should be decorated with mood lifting sceneries. Better to have a picture of the deity of patient's choice. This will generate great confidence in him. Arrangement should be made for soft music in the room. Recently a pillow has been introduced which is provided with a speaker. One can listen to music without disturbing others.

COPING WITH YOUR FEELINGS

Your emotions can affect your recovery and your risk of future cardiac events, so it's important to understand your feelings, recognize problems and get help if you need it

You may feel alone, scared or different from the person you were before you learned you had heart disease. And your emotions may be both negative and positive.

These feelings are very common — most heart patients have them. They may go away as you learn to **understand your heart condition** and manage it, but sometimes feelings such as depression may stay with you and require you to seek professional help.

FIGHT DEPRESSION

Major depression strikes about 20 percent of all people recovering from an attack, and another 20 percent suffer mild depression. The depression may fade over time, but the relief often turns out to be temporary. In any given year, one out of three long-term survivors of heart attack will slip into depression.

How dangerous is depression?
Severe depression can interfere with daily tasks just as surely as severe heart disease, sometimes to an even greater degree. And for heart patients, depression can even be deadly. Patients with major depression are three to four times as likely as other patients to die within six months of a heart attack. They are also more likely to suffer future heart attacks or return to the hospital for heart trouble.

Why are depression and heart disease such a dangerous mix? Part of the explanation lies in the body's reaction to stress. Depression can trigger the release of adrenaline and other "stress" hormones that have the potential to increase the heart rate, boost blood pressure, damage the inner lining of the heart muscle, and disrupt the heart's rhythm. The hormones can also speed the build up of fatty plaques in the arteries, setting the stage for another heart attack.

On a more basic level, depression can simply sap a person's will to fight heart disease. Severely depressed heart patients were less likely than non depressed patients to exercise regularly, give up smoking, eat a low-fat diet, or generally follow their doctor's advice.

How can I protect myself from depression?
First, be aware that clinical depression is not a normal part of recovery. Second, remember that cardiologists and primary care doctors may not realize their patients are depressed. To best protect yourself or a loved one from the burden of depression, you'll have to watch for the signs yourself. You should suspect depression if a person has five or more of the following symptoms for at least two weeks:

- frequent feelings of sadness or emptiness

- loss of interest in pleasurable activities

- strange eating or sleeping patterns

- excessive crying

- thoughts of suicide and death

- fatigue

- difficulty concentrating or remembering

- feelings of worthlessness or helplessness

- irritability

- unexplained aches and pains that don't respond to treatment

Are antidepressants safe for heart patients?
Tricyclic antidepressants, such as Elavil (amitriptyline), cause irregular, slow, or rapid heartbeat and other cardiac conduction disturbances, as well as a sudden drop in blood pressure and dizziness upon rising; these problems can be especially difficult to manage in patients with heart disease. Medications that depress serotonin levels such as Prozac (fluoxetine) represent a promising alternative to tricyclic drugs for the treatment of depression accompanying heart disease. In patients with stable heart disease, including patients with prior heart attacks and subsequent harm to the left ventricle, recent studies have shown that selective serotonin reuptake inhibitors (SSRIs) such as Pro-

zac caused few adverse events. They resulted in a clinically in-significant slowdown in heartbeat, and they didn't damage the function of the left ventricle. These drugs have been associated with occasional bleeding problems, however.

Besides seeing a doctor, what else may help me recover from depression?

You can do your part to overcome depression by getting regular exercise. Daily walks and a good exercise program, under your doctor's supervision, will improve your mood, boost your energy, and give you new strength to fight your disease. Of course, exercise will also strengthen your heart. And if you're battling depression and heart disease at the same time, you and your heart will need all of the strength you can get.

ORAL HEALTH AND HEART DISEASE

One possibility is that bacteria from mouth or products released by these bacteria travel through the blood stream to other parts of the body, where they damage lining of the blood vessels. It is commonly seen that patients with cardiovascular disease have elevated levels of periodontal bacteria. These bacteria contain lipopolysaccharides, toxins that can cause illness when released into the body.

This can be confirmed with the measurement of von Willebrand factor released from the cells lining the blood vessels. Studies are being made on a group of proteins known as acute phase response proteins. Levels of these proteins increases in chronic infections, injuries or other physical trauma. Scientists have found that C-reactive protein is a good indicator of second heart attack in cardiovascular patients. Other studies show that patients with periodontal infection have increased level of C - reactive protein, and that the levels drop when periodontal disease is treated. Three to four types of periodontal bacteria have also been identified in the vessel wall and in the fatty deposits in the vessels.

There may also be inflammatory response involving cytokines. When gum tissue becomes inflamed, white blood cells in the tissue start producing cytokines (small protein like signaling molecule). If the cytokines leak into the blood vessels, they may alter the lining of blood vessels and may facilitate the white cells to penetrate the vessel wall. This initiates the fatty accumulation on the vessel wall.

Smoking is a risk factor for oral health as well as for the heart. Smoking can increase the risk of periodontal bacteria entering the blood stream. Smoking also makes the blood vessel stickier which might facilitate the bacteria and/or their products attach to the vessel wall and cause damage.

It is found that people with periodontal disease are almost twice as likely to suffer from a coronary artery disease as compared to those without periodontal disease.

In one study Petra Saikki and colleagues at the University of Helsinki Finland found that 27 out of 40 patients who suffered heart attack and 15 out of 30 men with heart disease carried antibodies related to Chlamydia, which is more commonly known as gum disease. Compared to subjects who were free of heart disease only 7 out of 41 had such antibodies?

HIV AND HEART DISEASE

Those with HIV are also at risk of cardiovascular disease. Elevation in triglyceride level is a common observation in HIV positive patients along with high LDL (bad cholesterol) and low HDL (good cholesterol) which increase the likelihood of cardiovascular disease.

People suffering from HIV often have chronic inflammation of the arteries and veins perhaps due to long term exposure to the virus or due to therapies. Also inflamed arteries send signals to the body to send more T- cells but due to HIV their number is too short. Inflamed arteries are more likely to form plaque.

People with HIV are prone to kidney failure. Since kidneys help in stabilizing the blood pressure, they are linked to cardiovascular function. HIV virus can damage the tubules of the kidneys and affect the process of filtration. Some antiretroviral medicines can harm the kidneys; however, kidney failure is more common in patients not taking antiretroviral medication. Smoking should be stopped and diabetes monitored as both these factors enhance cardiovascular disease in HIV patients.

It is also important to note that HIV patients are living longer, and the risk for heart disease increases for both HIV-positive and HIV-negative people as they age. For this reason, everyone needs to be aware of cardiovascular risks and strategies to have healthy life.

FLU AND HEART

Flu is a common disease which occurs with change of weather when the influenza viruses multiply leaps and bound. People confuse colds and upper respiratory infections with flu. Flu in fact has much more severe symptoms like fever, chills, cough, and sore throat, runny or stuffy nose beside headaches, body aches and fatigue. The patient remains sick for few days. If you have heart disease, the flu may be much more severe leading to complications including bacterial pneumonia and worsening heart problem as the heart has to work hard to pump blood to the lungs. To avoid flu, one should try to remain away from the people who are sick. Hands should be washed frequently and kept away from the face. American College of cardiology recommends an annual flu vaccine in injection form to the patients suffering from cardiovascular disease before the flu season.

COLD WEATHER AND HEART

Cold weather has direct influence on our heart. Those who are susceptible mostly suffer heart attacks in winter. In winter months there is great variation in day and night temperatures. This disturbs the hormone balance. Hormones like cortisol and noradrenalin are affected, which may cause change in vascular activity. Low temperature may constrict coronary blood vessels as a result of which the heart muscle does not get proper blood supply. In cold weather body has to be kept warm and heart plays vital role in this temperature regulation. It has been found that in most of the cases of coronary heart disease acute temperature fluctuation and the extent of cold weather are mainly responsible.

There is slight variation throughout the year in factors like hemoglobin level, erythrocyte sedimentation rate (ESR), hematocrit value, percentage of coagulating platelets and fibrinolytic activity. During winter season, concentration of fibrinogen is high due to low temperature and high respiratory infection. Smoking is equally responsible for it. Due to low temperature the immune response is lowered which gives a chance to increase respiratory infection in heart disease patients. Otherwise also these patients are more prone to respiratory infection.

It is not clear whether heart patient deaths due to cold can be regulated. It is advised that such patients should keep their rooms warm with heater or blower. When going out one should wear enough warm clothing. Ears and face should be specially protected. Morning walk timing should be changed. It is better to go after sun rise. While exercising, care should be taken to exert gradually and the exercises which the body is unable to bear should be avoided.

HEART DISEASE AND TRAVEL

Those suffering from heart disease or those taking care of a heart patient generally limit their outings out of the fear of the ailment. If few simple precautions are taken, their travel may be quite smooth. For this one should have all the necessary things as used in routine. Here are the steps one should follow:

1.	Keep a copy of your prescription and pertinent medical record. This will help in case medicines are lost. Better to have it on your e-mail.

2.	Keep with you the phone number of your cardiologist.

3.	Tell your cardiologist about your destination. He may give you name and phone number of a cardiologist or a hospital there. Try to find out yourself the medical facilities there.

4.	Keep your medicines handy.

5.	Be aware of your insurance health covers and their requirements. Enquire about what emergency facility they may provide in case a problem arises.

6.	Need not to, if travelling to a higher altitude. Have enough fluid intake and balanced sodium consumption, if suffering from cardiomyopathy*. If suffering from coronary artery diseases watch for shortness of breath and other symptoms, which make you unstable. This may be due to low oxygen in the air. Avoid exertion.

7.   Sitting immobile can increase the risk of blood clots in legs. If someone has peripheral artery disease, the clot risk rises. So, avoid long bus or plane journeys. Walking around whenever possible will help.

* Pathological changes in the heart muscle.

HEART AND GENETIC COUNSELING

Some times in the family a child is born with congenital defect in the heart. It disturbs the family and the question arises "Why this occur to us" or any adult with congenital heart defect can ask "may this happen to us?" Genetic counseling is the facility which guides you before raising a family.

Q.   **How does genetic counseling work?**

A.   Experts of genetic counseling can ask a parent with genetic heart defect to undergo some tests which determine the chances of defect being inherited and can guide about further course. Sometimes blood samples of close relatives are also tested if they have heart problem.

Q.   **Who should have genetic counseling?**

A.   Parents with heart defects should go for counseling. They can know the cause of the defect. Both man and women should undergo testing because either one, if has a defect, may pass it on to the child. Genetic tests also give information about other diseases like deafness, psychiatric condition, liver disease or learning problem.

Q.   **When should one go for genetic counseling?**

A.   It is best for man and women to go for genetic counseling before marriage. If not, it is advised to go for counseling before getting pregnant, so that they understand the problem beforehand. By way of this, one knows if some special tests are to be taken during pregnancy. They can know if the fetus has inherited the defect or not by fetal echocardiography which is done by a paedriatic cardiologist.

 New developments in heart disease treatment

(1) **New enzyme complex developed from earthworms**.

In the coronary artery of a heart patient a clot is usually formed. Fibrin* is an important component of this clot which keeps binding all other components. Scientists have been trying for last ten years to isolate fibrin dissolving enzymes from several species of earthworm, including *Lumbricus, rubellas* and *Eisenia fetida.* A report published in Oxford University Press Journal in 2009 highlights the work of Prof. Edwin Cooper who has been successful in isolating lumbrokinase –a group of six novel proteolytic enzymes from the earthworm *Lumbricus rubellas.* This complex is capable of dissolving fibrin, decreasing fibrinogen (from which fibrin is formed), lowering blood viscosity and markedly reduce platelet aggregation. It is considered much superior to other such enzymes like streptokinase and urokinase as it dissolves fibrin and fibrinogen but hardly affects other important proteins such as plasminogen and albumin. Toxicological experiments have not found any adverse effects on liver and kidney function due to lumbrokinase. It has no negative effect on blood glucose and fats.

(2) **Computer model depicts effect of medicines on the heart**

Scientists have developed a computer model that predicts the effect of anti-arrhythmic medicines on the heart. It confirms the results of experiments done on animals and humans. It is hoped that in future the medicines would be tested without time consuming animal experimentation. Also, millions of molecules could be tested in a short time and with little expenditure. The study is based on the fact that in the heart electrical impulses are generated by the flow of charged molecules or ions across the cell membrane. Arrhythmia (irregular heart beat) occurs when flow across the membrane becomes defective. Anti-arrhythmic drugs regularize the flow of ions. A wrong dose of medicine can make the symptoms worse which may lead to death.

* An insoluble protein formed during clotting of blood which impedes the flow of blood

In the computer model scientists used equations to represent the opening and closing of the channels in the cell membrane that allow the ions to flow across the membrane generating impulses. Researchers can feed the medicine and the dose and the model will predict what effect the drug has on the heart.

Q.   Is it possible to predict occurrence of heart disease?

A.   Heart disease is caused as cumulative effects of many factors like genetic, life style, eating habits, general activity and behavioral make- up of the person. Although it is difficult to predict heart disease, family history and behavioral pattern can give some indications. Those with a heart disease family history can expect the disease and therefore, should have regular checkup. Earlier studies based on the history of heart patients have found that people who are very assertive and ambitious may have heart problem. Such people try to be on every committee, they become assertive with blowing their fist on the table. They are time conscious and see the watch 16 times in one hour. Worry is another great cause of heart problem. Chartered Accountants who have to file tax statements in a time schedule are often overloaded with work when due date is approaching. This may lead to heart problem due to worry and over exertion.

Formation of plaque in the coronary artery is associated with inflammation. C-reactive protein (CRP) is a sensitive protein. Increase in its level when measured with highly sensitive assays can predict risk of myocardial infarction. Use of CRP level determination for screening of general population is not recommended.

Inflammation in oral diseases is linked with coronary heart disease, and since oral diseases are quite common, this could be used for public health screening.

(3)   Heart attack prediction

A new coin size device has been introduced which will predict the onset of a heart attack. It is implanted near the left shoulder to monitor the electric activities of the heart muscle. When there is an abnormal pattern, the device detects it and vibrates. As a result of it, a pager produces signal by alarm and light.

(4)   A new stent

Till recent past veins harvested from the legs were used to make new channels from the clogged artery, which may last for about 15 years. Dr. Michael Kutryk of Toronto University has developed a new type of stent which is coated with an antibody that captures naturally occurring endothelial cells present in our circulatory system, which help in the healing of our arteries. Further modification of it is a biodegradable one in which besides healing, the endothelial cells also prevent the arteries from constricting. Dr.Kutryk says, "In future we will put in a biodegradable stent that contains healthy artery promoting compound. As the stent is dissolving, it will release compounds in to the vessel wall to accelerate the natural healing process." After a month or so the artery will be completely normal. The new stent is in preclinical evaluation and will be put to a human trial soon.

(5)   Valve replacement

Till recently valve replacement was done through open heart surgery. Dr. Eric Horlick, an interventional cardiologist of Peter Munk cardiac Centre at Toronto General Hospital has pioneered a much less invasive procedure. In this procedure the heart is not stopped. It continues to beat. A catheter is inserted in the vein in the groin with a clip to repair the valve. It is taken up to the heart with the help of a 3D guidance system and the clip is fixed at proper place. This procedure is very important for the people who have other major problems of the heart. Dr Horlick has also performed pulmonary and aortic valve replacements.

(6)   A new drug

On the basis of an international trial on 13,655 heart patients, it is claimed that those who were taking, aspirin, beta blockers and cholesterol lowering drugs did better when they also took a new drug perindopril. It is an ACE inhibitor which dilates blood vessels and brings down blood pressure. It reduced incidence of heart attack and death by 20 percent.

(7)   A new blood thinner

A new blood thinner fondaparinux has been introduced by a Canadian team. It is found to be better at preventing heart attacks and strokes as compared to the prevalent drugs. Good thing is that it does not cause gastrointestinal bleeding and it is cheaper.

(8)   ECG/CT

By making use of ECG and computed tomography a new technique has been developed for arrhythmic beating of the heart, which will give better information about the beating of the different parts of the heart.

(9)   Stem cells

Stem cells are sometimes called as generic cells of the body which have the ability to differentiate into most of the cell types of the body. They can repair the damaged parts of the body. Dr. Joshua Hare of Interdisciplinary Stem Cell Institute at American University of Miami in 2009 proved that infusing stem cells in heart attack patients is safe and that the treatment helped the patients in recovering. Dr. Hare's team worked on 45 cardiac patients who were quite weak and bed ridden. After treatment with stem cells, they were able to walk reasonable distance.

(10)   Music heals the heart

According to the American Heart Association people who listen to their favorite music frequently for few months, show a tendency of lowering their blood pressure to the tune of low salt diet or losing five kilo weight.

(11)   A new cholesterol bursting injection

A new cholesterol bursting injection, which could save the lives of millions, is being hailed as a potential breakthrough in battle against heart attacks and strokes. The volunteers had three quarter of artery blockage, but with the new drug it was all cleared.

(12)   Weight loss

Researchers of Leed Metropolitan University have carried out a study and found that men who attend slimming classes could manage to shed twice as much weight when there are no women around. For the study, 62 overweight men from the West Midlands attended weekly weight watchers' meetings without any women. Around two thirds of the men completed the course and 77% of them lost at least 5% of their body weight. Some shed more than 10%. According to lead researcher Professor Steven Robertson, "A lot of men said that they felt a very female dominated meeting might put them off contributing or taking things which were important for them." It is likely that some of the men are bashful about discussing their chubby bodies in front of women.

CONVERSATION WITH YOUR DOCTOR

When someone in your family is suffering from tiredness on walking short distance, you must consult a cardiologist. If there is discomfort and it subsides in five minutes, still go to the doctor. Don't be panicky, but be more composed and attend to the needs of the patient. The chief attendant should only discuss with the doctor as the latter will not be able to make understand everybody. The doctor will suggest some tests. Mostly people do not discuss with the doctor, and many questions remain unanswered. Be free to discuss. Ask the doctor as to what the actual stage of the disease is, what precautions are to be taken and what meals should be taken, should the tests be repeated. Tell the doctor what drugs the patient has been taking. On the basis of the condition of the patient the doctor may prescribe some medicines or may ask to go for angiography. The drugs prescribed may be cholesterol level decreasing drugs, low dose aspirin to keep the platelets from sticking together and medicines to reduce the heart rate and blood pressure. Ask the doctor if they are brand name medicines or generic medicines. The latter are cheaper. Besides the medication, the doctor should tell you about control of other risk factors like inactivity, oily food, diabetes and obesity. Ask the doctor how frequently to meet so that the he can have a track record of the disease. Discuss with him the emergency plan, as to where to take the patient if he feels more discomfort and what medicine should be taken at that time. Know more about angiography and other tests before they are performed. At the time of doctors round the chief attendant should be present. If he is unable to understand anything, he should make it clear with the doctor. The attendants can also keep a track record of the patient on the basis of the patient chart available on the bed side. If the drugs are showing any side effects, it should be reported to the doctor. If operation is suggested, ask the doctor about the risk if the operation is delayed. On the basis of the reports available second opinion may be obtained to ascertain the stage of the disease and line of treatment. Always keep the prescription and medicines with you when going to hospital or travelling.

STEM CELLS

Until recently there was nothing which could repair the damaged site of the heart; which normally stays as a scar and leaves the patient with difficulty in breathing, increased weakness and inability to take strain. Now when a patient suffering from heart attack arrives at a hospital the doctors restore the blood flow by removing the blockage so that no further damage is done to the heart. Some patients need transplant while 50% have heart so weak, they die. Now doctors can repair the damaged sites to the extent that the weakened heart becomes almost normal working again. It pumps blood closer to the way it did before the heart attack. This is possible through the use of stem cells.

Stem cells are embryonic cells which can differentiate into other types of cells. They can be recovered by three ways:

(1) From the tissue of the embryo. They are known as embryonic stem cells.

(2) Chord stem cells: recovered from the placenta at the time of delivery.

(3) Adult stem cells: recovered from the bone marrow.

When chord is cut, the cord blood is collected. This contains hematopoietic stem cells; mesenchymal stem cells and embryonic like stem cells. Chord was generally discarded but now the parents like to deposit it in the stem cell bank for future use. Recent researches have opened new avenues for repairing body organs. Now tissue specific progenitor cells have also been identified. The adult heart contains cardiac stem cells that are self-renewing and able to produce identical daughter cells and are multipotent i.e., they can differentiate into cardiac muscle cells,

cells forming blood vessels, smooth muscle cells and endothelial cells which form the inner lining of the heart. At the American heart Association session in October 2012 Dr. Roberto Bollis of the University of Louisville and Dr.Piero Anversa of Brigham and Women Hospital, Boston presented data on the ground breaking research in the use of autologous adult stem cells in patients who had heart attack. The data showed that after two years, all the patients receiving stem cell therapy showed improvement in heart function. As a result of heart attack the capacity of the left ventricle to send blood to body parts (LVEF –Left Ventricular Ejection Factor) is reduced, because some part of the heart muscle is dead and a scar of connective tissue fibers is left. Normal LVEF is 50 or higher while all the patients in this study had LVEF less than 40. Patients treated with stem cells showed an overall 12.9 absolute units increase in LVEF. No adverse effects were observed. Moreover, MRI showed regeneration of heart muscle. Another study made at Minneapolis has shown that stem cell therapy is safe and there is now a base line in terms of quantity of stem cells, type of stem cells and severity of heart attack. Since the cells are from the same patient there is little chance of rejection problems that often occur when tissue is transplanted from another person. Researchers at Cedar-Sinai Heart Institute and the John Hopkins University found that patients had significantly less scarring of the heart muscle after six months of treatment. Also, there was considerable increase in healthy heart muscle. The doctors experienced a drawback in this procedure, that the patient undergoes painful bone marrow harvests. The harvested cells are prepped which sometimes can take weeks. Dr. Mare Penn a cardiologist of Summa Health System at Akron has been collecting stem cells ahead of time from young healthy donors and stored in a freezer so that they can be used when the patient arrives. The results show that the heart of the patients so treated worked as normal hearts at least for a year.

A team of John Hopkins researchers have identified a single

protein molecule *p190RhoGAP* which may have key role in transforming stem cells into cardiac muscle tissue or blood vessel. They found that changing the surface on which the harvested cells grow would affect the cells' development. When cells were grown on surface resembling the rigidity of the heart tissue, the stem cells grew faster and formed blood vessels. In plastic and glass dishes the cell population grew far less. Dr.Levchenko of the research team described the *p190RhoGAP* molecule as the master regulator molecule. When its level was decreased the cell, growth was increased. When the level was increased, more of the muscle cells were formed. When this molecule was completely removed, special heart – matched surfaces were not required. The stem cells started to form blood vessels even on glass. Dr Kshitiz the co-worker of Dr. Levchenko says, "This single protein can control the cells, shape, how fast they divide how they become blood vessel cells and how they start forming a blood vessel network. How it performed all of these myriad tasks that require hundreds of other proteins to act in a complex interplay was an interesting mystery to address, and that rarely occurs in biology. It was like a molecular symphony being played in time, with each beat placed right at the moment before another melody has to start".

MAKING LIFESTYLE CHANGES

After a heart attack one must make necessary changes in his life style. He must think about the factors that made him suffer a heart attack and if not corrected may slow recovery.

They may be:

A Lazy life-- lack of exercise

Stress-- being over ambitious

Uncared diabetes

Poor eating habits -- no consideration for calories.

Eating oily food.

Smoking and tobacco chewing

Excessive alcohol drinking

Irregular and insufficient sleep

Uncared high blood pressure

If these factors are taken care of, the risk of another heart attack and stroke can be minimized.

Making life style changes may look hard, but it is necessary and rewarding. It's usually easier to change when other people are there to show you how to make changes. One should be smart enough to bring about life style changes by oneself and not as a compulsion. By adopting changes in lifestyle, you plan your future where you can enjoy best quality of life.

Cholesterol management

Your ideal cholesterol depends upon your age, gender, weight and history of heart disease. Some people do have family history of having high cholesterol level. They should regularly monitor their lipid profile. People who have heart disease or had a heart attack should maintain their LDL level below 70mg/dl. It may be managed by adopting habit of taking simple and nutritious food, regular exercise and meditation. Avoid saturated fats (cream, butter, ghee, animal fat, vanaspati, etc.), Reduce total intake of calories to keep weight under control. Add more polyunsaturated fatty acids (omega 3 and omega 6 fatty acids) in your diet as they have cholesterol lowering effect.

Exercise

If you were sedentary and sluggish before, you can't afford to remain the same. You need to be active, because exercise helps you on several fronts. It strengthens the heart, burns calories and raises your stamina so that you can lead a normal life. Regular exercise has also been linked to better mental health. Physical activity is used in the treatment of depression—a common problem for heart patients. Patients, who just had heart attacks or open-heart surgery, may wonder how much exertion their heart can take. Professionals may help at this stage. A cardiologist or a physiotherapist tells you what exercises you can undertake at different stages, depending upon your physical strength and other medical factors. Afterwards, it is up to you to follow the instructions and schedule exercise in your daily routine.

When we go to gym, our specific body organs get exercise. Walking is considered best exercise as it helps all the body organs. Thirty-minute walk is sufficient for heart patients. It should be initial five minutes warming, followed by twenty-minute brisk walk and five minutes slow down. Since people do not have much time, they prefer to walk on tread mill at home. It is difficult to distinguish between tread mill walking and open-air walking, however, in tread mill walking one does not experience the opposite current of air outside. It is, therefore better to keep tread mill at a little inclination. This gives extra load to your heart and makes it like walking in open air with opposite wind. Another factor involved is that walking on tread mill gives lesser impact on knees as compared to walking on the pavement. So, you do not build the same muscular endurance as one gets outdoors.

Quit smoking

Smoking has both short- and long-term effects on the body. Recent study suggests that smoking may bring about changes in genes paving ways for the serious diseases like cancer. Quitting at any age will benefit you but earlier you quit better it is. Two to three, months after quitting, your circulation and lung function improve. One to nine months after quitting coughing and shortness of breath decreases. Cilia in the respiratory tract return to normal function, which makes it easier to clear mucous from the lungs and the trachea and reduce the risk of infection by one year of quitting. Your risk of cardiovascular disease is reduced to half. Five years after quitting risk is equal to that of a nonsmoker. Ten years after quitting risk of lung, mouth, throat esophageal, bladder and pancreatic cancer is greatly reduced. Besides this you add up to your personality by way of better smelling breath, better teeth, better taste of food and get rid of smoky smell from your clothes, hair and your room.

Stress

People are at large not aware of how much stress may damage their heart. An altogether changed mindset has to be adopted. Plan your life free of tiring responsibilities. If need be, a new profession may be taken with rather more free time to relax and take care of your heart. If you encounter any problem in managing stress, your doctor or a psychotherapist should be consulted.

Diet

Acquiring a taste for healthy food may be the easiest and wisest lifestyle change to make. Breaking the smoking habit may be the hardest. After a heart attack you'll have to cut back on food that is bad for your heart and arteries. Mind your food- always keep a record of what you have eaten throughout the day. This will help you monitor your diet. Watch closely your intake of alcohol, sugary drinks, fast food, and salt. If you often suffer with acidity, minimize your sugar intake.

Take minimum quantity of salt as it may help in raising blood pressure. Most of the vegetables have sufficient salt which is enough for our body functions. Include more vegetables and fruits in your diet. When you are invited to a party, it's always better to have your regular meal at home before going to party. Or else in the party have more salad, eat patiently with proper chewing. Avoid starters. Select the items that are not fried or have minimum oil.

The range of heart-healthy food in the market is much better than it once was. You have plenty of options. Heart-healthy recipes and cookbooks are easy to find, on the web or at bookstores. You should read labels on prepared food more carefully. You may have to adjust your taste buds a bit. For the latest research and recommendations on healthy eating, go to the American Heart Association Web site, www.americanheart.org, scroll to "Healthy Lifestyle" on the home page and click "Diet & Nutrition."

Losing weight—

Some people, who want to slash down their weight, cut their diet as it helps in quickly losing weight, but it is not proper method because when you stop restricting your diet, you again put on weight. In fact, when you go for dieting your body becomes accustomed to that amount of food and it functions at a lower metabolic rate. When you stop dieting and take normal amount of food, the extra amount of food is stored as fat. If you are overweight and want to lose some, the trick is to set goals which can be achieved. Losing weight at a rate of about 0.5 to 1.0 kg per week is right.

You may find many advertisements all around you offering miraculous products which may help you lose weight, but the question remains, whether they do help you?   Some may be dangerous, subjecting your body to lack of nourishment that it needs. People are committing mistakes in taking diet for normal living and for losing weight. Eating a healthy, balanced diet is essential for good health and cutting out entire food groups is harmful, so it is important to eat a range of foods from the five main food groups (carbohydrates, fats, proteins, minerals and vitamins). Try to eat less fat. Fat has more than twice the calories of carbohydrates and protein. So, remember to satisfy your hunger with bread, potatoes, rice and pasta when trying to lose excess weight. Try to find low-fat alternatives to creamy sauces and choose cooking methods that keep the overall fat content low. Don't forget that even a small portion of healthy pasta has a lot of calories. Serving food on smaller plates will reduce intake to some extent. Although diets such as the Atkins's diet advocate cutting out fruit and vegetables, it's important to include at least five portions of these in your daily diet. Fruit and vegetables are rich in essential vitamins, minerals and fiber. Steamed, boiled or raw, they are both filling and low in calories

Behavior towards family

After a heart attack the patient becomes weak and irritating. One should understand the prevalent conditions at the moment. Many people undergo depression after heart attack or bypass surgery. It has to be taken easy, as it is a matter of few days. Gradually the health improves and these symptoms disappear. The patient should control anger and irritation on minor things. Also, he should wisely deal with the family members and friends who seldom try to overdo things for him. People may give undue advice and suggestions which need not be given heed unless cleared by your cardiologist. During the period of recovery, the patient should strengthen bondage with the family members having a positive attitude. This enhances recovery.

Try to be in contact with your friends. According to the study done at University of North Carolina, one should be quite social. Death rate is more in those having poor social contacts as compared to those who have good social contacts. Meeting friends is very helpful in the recovery period. If you are unable to meet the friend, talk to them on phone for at least for ten minutes.

It is likely that when you are recovering at home you sit more than two hours before TV. Try to avoid sitting in front of TV for long durations. It may reduce the rate of recovery. If you are very much fond of seeing a program, get up and walk after sitting for an hour or two.

Help some one

It is well known that those who help others are happier. Find out someone who is in need. Help him by money, accompanying, advising or other means. It will bring in you positivity and a sense of usefulness in the society. By way of it you can have social circle and win friends. Play cards with them and ward off the stress. Social engagements in advancing age are as good as lowering cholesterol or blood pressure.

Q.   Is alcohol good for the heart?

A.   Wine and other alcoholic beverages are heart friendly; the impact lasts long after the alcohol leaves your body system. Studies have shown that consumption of moderate amount of alcohol (80ml) can improve your HDL level which lowers heart disease risk both in men and women. Many studies have shown that a small glass of wine a day is good for your heart. Red wine contains an antioxidant resveratrol which is found in grapes, mulberries and pea nuts. Studies made on animals suggest that this antioxidant improves exercise endurance as well as protects against obesity and insulin resistance which may lead to diabetes. Heavy drinking is bad for your heart. If you drink to deal with stress, learn healthier ways to relax.

Q. Is coconut oil good for heart?

A. Coconut oil is a member of saturated fat group which are considered bad for the heart health but recent studies have reported that coconut oil in limited amount is good for the heart. A study made in Brazil in 2009 on women showed that it decreased the waist line, increased HDL cholesterol and improved the ratio of HDL and LDL. It is evident in the populations where coconut is routinely used in cooking; the incidence of heart ailments is low. It is advised to limit saturated fat to 10% of your daily calorie intake. For this coconut oil or milk should be preferred.

Q. Is chocolate good for heart?

A. Recent finding, that is sure to delight many of us with a sweet tooth claim that chocolate consumption may be associated with a 33 percent decrease in the risk of developing heart disease. While other factors are, much more important for a healthy heart like exercise and proper eating this study has given a nice reprieve to chocolates. Other studies show that dark chocolate is much better as it contains more cocoa which is rich in flavanols and polyphones. New research at the Faculty of Life Sciences (LIFE) at the University of Copenhagen – shows that dark chocolate is far more filling than milk chocolate, lessening our craving for sweet, salty and fatty foods. In other words, eating dark chocolate may be an efficient way to keep your weight down over the holidays.

We have known for a long time that it is healthier to eat dark chocolate, but now scientists at the Department of Human Nutrition at LIFE, University of Copenhagen, have found that dark chocolate also gives more of a feeling of satiety than milk chocolate.

To compare the effects of dark and milk chocolate on both appetite and subsequent calorie intake, 16 young and healthy men of normal weight who all liked both dark and milk chocolate took part in a so-called crossover experiment. This meant that they reported for two separate sessions, the first time testing the dark chocolate, and the second time the milk chocolate.

They had all fasted for 12 hours beforehand and were offered 100g of chocolate, which they consumed in the course of 15 minutes. The calorific content was virtually the same for the milk and dark chocolate.

During the following 5 hours, participants were asked to register their appetite every half hour, i.e., their hunger, satiety, craving for special foods and how they liked the chocolate.

Two and a half hours after eating the chocolate, participants were offered pizza. They were instructed to eat until they felt comfortably satiated. After the meal, the individual's calorie intake was registered.

The results were significant. The calorie intake at the subsequent meal where they could eat as much pizza as they liked was 15 per cent lower when they had eaten dark chocolate beforehand.

The participants also stated that the plain chocolate made them feel less like eating sweet, salty or fatty foods.

So apart from providing us with the healthier fatty acids and many antioxidants, dark chocolate can be considered a healthy food item.

Exercise —most people work on a two-pronged approach i.e., low calorie diet and increased physical activity. Under some conditions the physical activity is less useful particularly when you are just starting to increase your activity. Some people take enough hard stress in the beginning which may be troublesome. Similarly, people take up hard exercise after a gap of a week or so for two three days. A relatively unfit person running hard for 10 minutes a couple of times a week is unlikely to lose much weight – and in fact, it could even be dangerous.

According to the UK Department of Health, you need to do at least 30 minutes of moderate exercise, such as brisk walking or swimming on five or more days a week. If you're overweight or obese, you will probably need to do more than this. Moderate activity should increase your heart beats and make you feel slightly warm and a little out of breath.

THORACIC AORTIC ANEURISM

Aorta is the largest blood vessel arising from the heart, takes a turn and runs entire length supplying various organs up to the posterior abdomen. It then divides into two and supplies blood to the legs. Sometimes the wall of the aorta bulges. This condition is known as aortic aneurism. This is weak area of the aorta. Aneurism may occur anywhere along the length of the aorta. Generally, it occurs in the patients who have had a heart stenting or have undergone by-pass surgery. The weakened area may start leaking giving rise to internal bleeding. Sometimes it is fatal. In November 2011 three cases were reported from Medanta Medicity at Gurgaon (India) who were all above 70 years and had undergone by-pass surgery 10-12 years ago and had normal health. All of them complained of progressive hoarseness of voice. The ENT surgeons could not detect any local pathology. CT scan of the chest revealed localized enlargement in the arch of the aorta, which was pressing the nerve innervating the vocal cords causing hoarseness. Incidence of aneurism is as high as 10% in the population of who have undergone stenting or by-pass surgery. It appears to be more in men than in women; however, women with aneurism have a higher risk of rupturing of the blood vessel. Aneurism may be corrected by (1) opening the chest or abdomen to replace the damaged part of the blood vessel with an artificial tube or (2) by placing a covered stent graft inside the affected blood vessel to prevent them from dilating and eventually rupturing. With this treatment the hoarseness also subsides within eight weeks.

Factors responsible for this ailment are:

(1)   Aortic thoracic aneurism mostly occurs in patients suffering from diabetes aged 60 or more.
(2)   Longer is the period of smoking or chewing tobacco greater is the risk.
(3)   High blood pressure damages the blood vessels, raising the chances of developing aneurism.
(4)   Atherosclerosis (building up of plaques in the blood vessels) can damage   the lining of the blood vessel, increasing the risk.
(5)   People who have a family history of aortic aneurism are at increased risk.
Doctors suggest that patients should be aware that those who suffer from sudden and progressive hoarseness of voice with an ENT specialist unable to find the cause could be suffering from aneurism and should contact a cardiovascular surgeon.

ARTIFICIAL HEART

When all other treatments have failed and both the ventricles are not able to pump blood to the vital organs, then the need of an artificial heart arises. It may be required for a short time till the original heart becomes efficient enough. If the patient's heart can't recover, the artificial heart works till he gets a heart transplant. If no other options are available the artificial heart can stay permanently.

An artificial heart is a pump, something like an extra ventricle which takes over the function of pumping the blood to body organs. Technically it is known as 'ventricular assist device' (VAD). A VAD is made of plastic and metal having a small pumping chamber, lined by special material which does not allow blood to clot. It may be put inside or outside body of the patient depending on the type of artificial heart being used. If the left ventricle is very weak, it is attached to the left ventricle and the aorta. It is then known as 'left ventricular assist device' (LVAD). If support is needed by the right ventricle, then it is attached between right ventricle and the pulmonary artery and is called 'right ventricular assist device (RVAD).

If support is needed by both the ventricles then both LVAD and RVAD are used.

Q. How does an artificial heart work?

A. Blood collected in the right ventricle from the right atrium is pumped into the pulmonary artery, and that collected in the left ventricle is pumped into the aorta.

An artificial heart is powered either by compressed air or by electricity. It is connected with the help of a thin cable to a control console which regulates its function. A console can be large enough kept on wheels and kept by the side of the patient or it may move with the patient when he walks. It may also be small   with batteries and worn by the patient on a belt.

An artificial heart is generally used for a waiting period till the patient gets a transplant or if the patient is not suitable for heart transplant, a total artificial heart is used which can work for several years. Matthew green resident of Cambridge-share is the first person to receive the artificial heart. According to Dr. Steven Tsui of Pepworth Hospital, 40-year-old Green was suffering from right ventricular myopathology, a disease in which the heart may stop working any time and the patient dies. He could not wait for donor heart. Therefore, this artificial heart implant was necessary. Greens artificial heart is operated by a portable driver fitted on his back. This heart serves the role of both ventricles and heart valves. The device provides a blood flow up to 9.5 liters', eliminating symptoms and effects of heart failure, now he can have a normal life till he gets a natural donor heart.

Recently a patient in France got transplantation of a new type of heart which will work like a normal heart. This is manufactured by a biomedical firm Carmat. This device is intended to replace a real heart for as many as five years, unlike the above-described artificial hearts that were invented mainly for temporary use. It is a self-contained unit implanted in the chest of the patient, uses soft biomaterials and an array of sensors to mimic the contractions of the heart. This product provides long term solution to bridge the wait for a donor heart and enable patients to return home and may resume work, in place of waiting in the hospital. The patient has to wear a belt of lithium batteries to power the heart. At present its size is suitable for the men, however heart suitable for women is also being prepared.

REFERENCES

www.bupa.co.uk/individuals/health-information/directory/d/
diet-crash-diets 2/2

www.bupa.co.uk/individuals/health-information/directory/d/
diet-crash-diets 1/2

Eating *to Lower Your High Blood Cholesterol,* (pamphlet), pp. 4-8;
Hopkins, Nigel J., John W. Mayne, and John R. Hudson. *The Numbers You Need,* p. 84; Wyngaarden, James B., and Lloyd **H.** Smith. Cecil *Textbook of Medicine,* p. 1208.

Sources: Dull, Charles E. *Modern Physics,* p. 243; Ontario Science Center Staff. *Foodworks: Over One Hundred Science Activities and Fascinating Facts That Explore the Magic of Food,* p. 72

www.ehow.com

http://wzen.ask.com

http://www.webmd.com/diet/features/estimated-calorie-re-quiremen

http://nutrition.about.com/library/bl_nutrition_guide_men.htm

Med India: Fish Oil and Yeast Rice Effectively Control Bad Cholesterol: Study

"Natural Solutions" magazine; The Anti Inflammation Diet; Catherine Guthrie; December 2003

Mayo Clinic: Omega-3 Fatty Acids, Fish Oil, Alpha-linolenic Acid

American Heart Aassociation: Fish, Levels of Mercury and Omega-3 Fatty Acids

Read more: http://www.livestrong.com/article/110965-fish-oil-protect-heart/#ixzz24x9NaLBV

References

·   Gupta R, Prakash H. Association of dietary ghee intake with coronary heart disease and risk factor prevalence in rural males. J Indian Med Assoc 1997;95(3):67-9, 83. 1997.

·   Kumar MV, Sambaiah K, Lokesh BR. Effect of dietary ghee--the anhydrous milk fat, on blood and liver lipids in rats. J Nutr Biochem 1999;10(2):96-104. 1999.

·   Kumar MV, Sambaiah K, Lokesh BR. Hypocholesterolemic effect of anhydrous milk fat ghee is mediated by increasing the secretion of biliary lipids. J Nutr Biochem 2000;11(2):69-75. 2000.

·   Nestel PJ, Chronopulos A, Cehun M. Dairy fat in cheese raises LDL cholesterol less than that in butter in mildly hypercholesterolaemic subjects. Eur J Clin Nutr 2005 Sep;59(9):1059-63. 2005.

·   Niranjan TG, Krishnakantha TP. Effect of dietary ghee--the anhydrous milk fat on lymphocytes in rats. Mol Cell Biochem 2001;226(1-2):39-47. 2001.

·   Prattala RS, Groth MV, Oltersdorf US, et al. Use of butter and cheese in 10 European countries: a case of contrasting educational differences. Eur J Public Health 2003 Jun;13(2):124-32. 2003.

·   Shankar SR, Bijlani RL, Baveja T, et al. Effect of partial replacement of visible fat by ghee (clarified butter) on serum lipid profile. Indian J Physiol Pharmacol 2002;46(3):355-60. 2002.

·   Shankar SR, Yadav RK, Ray RB, et al. Serum lipid response to introducing ghee as a partial replacement for mustard oil in the diet of healthy young Indians. Indian J Physiol Pharmacol 2005 Jan;49(1):49-56. 2005.

- Singh RB, Niaz MA, Ghosh S, et al. Association of trans fatty acids (vegetable ghee) and clarified butter (Indian ghee) intake with higher risk of coronary artery disease in rural and urban populations with low fat consumption. Int J Cardiol 1996 Oct 25;56(3):289-98; discussion 299-300. 1996.

- Trevisan M, Krogh V, Freudenheim J, et al. Consumption of olive oil, butter, and vegetable oils and coronary heart disease risk factors. The Research Group ATS-RF2 of the Italian National Research Council. JAMA 1990, Vol. 263 No. 5: 688 - 692. 1990.

- Yellowlees WW. Milk, butter, and heart disease. Lancet 1991 Apr 27;337(8748):1041-2. 1991.

1] Caraka- Samhita. Translated by Sharma RK and Bhagwan Dash, 7th ed. Varanasi, India Chowkhama Sanskrit Series Office, 2002: 537 Sutrasthana 27/232)

[2] Caraka- Samhita. Translated by Sharma RK and Bhagwan Dash, 7th ed. Varanasi, India Chowkhama Sanskrit Series Office, 2002: 500 Sharirasthana 8/46

[3] Caraka- Samhita. Translated by Sharma RK and Bhagwan Dash, 7th ed. Varanasi, India Chowkhama Sanskrit Series Office, 2002: 532 Sutrasthana 27/217-224

[4] Kulkarni PH. Ayurvedic Aahar, Pune, India: Ayurvedic Education series, 1998: 110

[5] Caraka- Samhita. Translated by Sharma RK and Bhagwan Dash, 7th ed. Varanasi, India Chowkhama Sanskrit Series Office, 2002 Chikitsasthana 15/201

[6] Vijayalakshmi B; Kumara Swamy BV; Shantha TR: Ayurvedic rationale of the Southern Indian vegetable soup Saaru or rasam.

Ancient Science of Life Vol 17 (3), January 1998: 207-213

[7] Caraka- Samhita. Translated by Sharma RK and Bhagwan Dash, 7th ed. Varanasi, India Chowkhama Sanskrit Series Office, 2002: 532 Chikitsasthana 28/ 242-249

[8] Reddy Ramachandra K. Bhaisajya Kalpana Vijnanam, Varanasi, India: Chaukhambha Sanskrit Bhawan, 1998: 363

[9] Ng CH, Qiang Yao X, Huang Y, Chen ZY: **Oxidised cholesterol is more hypercholesterolaemic and atherogenic than non-oxidised cholesterol in hamsters.**Br J Nutr. 2008 Apr;99(4):749-55. Epub 2007 Oct 5

[10] Jacobson MS: Cholesterol Oxides in Indian Ghee: Possible cause of unexplained high risk of atherosclerosis in Indian immigrant populations. The Lancet, 1987, September 19: 656-658

[11] Nath BS and Rama Murthy MK: Cholesterol in Indian Ghee. The Lancet, 1998, July 2: 39

[12] Kumar MV, Sambaiah, K, Lokesh BR: The anhydrous milk fat, ghee, lowers serum prostaglandins and secretion of leukotrienes by rat peritoneal macrophages. Prostaglandins, Leukotrines and Essential Fatty Acids, 1999, Vol 61, Issue 4: 249-254

[13] Kumar MV, Sambaiah K, Lokesh BR: Hypocholesterolemia effect of anhydrous milk fat ghee is mediated by increasing the secretion of biliary lips. Journal of Nutritional Biochemistry, 2000, 11: 69-75

[14] Singh RB, Niaz MA, Ghosh S, Beegom R, Rastogi V, Sharma JP, Dube GK: Association of trans fatty acids (vegetable ghee) and clarified butter (Indian ghee) intake with higher risk of coronary artery disease in rural and urban populations with low fat con-

sumption. International Journal of Cardiology, Vol. 56, Issue 3: 289-298.

[15] Erasmus U. Fats that heal, Fats that kill, Canada: Alive Books, 1993: 118

[16] Reddy Ramachandra K. Bhaisajya Kalpana Vijnanam, Varanasi, India: Chaukhambha Sanskrit Bhawan, 1998: 365

[17] Erasmus U. Fats that heal, Fats that kill, Canada: Alive Books, 1993: 230

[18] Erasmus U. Fats that heal, Fats that kill, Canada: Alive Books, 1993: 124